RECENT ADVANCES IN HEMATOLOGY RESEARCH

HEMATOMAS

TYPES, TREATMENTS AND HEALTH RISKS

RECENT ADVANCES IN HEMATOLOGY RESEARCH

Additional books in this series can be found on Nova's website under the Series tab.

Additional E-books in this series can be found on Nova's website under the E-book tab.

PUBLIC HEALTH IN THE 21ST CENTURY

Additional books in this series can be found on Nova's website under the Series tab.

Additional E-books in this series can be found on Nova's website under the E-book tab.

RECENT ADVANCES IN HEMATOLOGY RESEARCH

HEMATOMAS

TYPES, TREATMENTS AND HEALTH RISKS

MISAEL F. GARZA SALAZAR
AND
ARACELI RUIZ MENDOZA
EDITORS

Nova Science Publishers, Inc.
New York

For permission to use material from this book please contact us:
Telephone 631-231-7269; Fax 631-231-8175
Web Site: http://www.novapublishers.com

Additional color graphics may be available in the e-book version of this book.

Library of Congress Cataloging-in-Publication Data

ISBN: 978-1-61942-385-5

Published by Nova Science Publishers, Inc. † New York

Contents

Preface

This book presents topical research in the study of the types, treatments and health risks associated with hematomas. Topics discussed include the physiotherapeutic treatments of hematomas; cerebrospinal hematoma; infected hematomas; the etiology of pelvic hematomas; intracranial hematomas in pediatric patients; massive retroperitoneal hematoma following vaginal correction of vault prolapse and retropharyngeal hematomas.

Chapter I - Physiotherapy is a health care science steadily evolving in its fundaments as well as in its methodology. The way to tackle the treatment of hematomas has been significantly improved, even if it essentially follows the same basic principles. In the same way, the physiotherapy and physical exercise prescribed for patients with hemophilia, must take into account several transcendent aspects.

In order to develop an efficient and specific physiotherapy, the first aspect to be taken into account is the identification and knowledge of the problem, in this case, the hematomas. The second aspect will be to establish an order of priorities and objectives, which will lead the chronology of the therapeutic actions, the effects of which must also be considered.

Hematomas can be classified according to their nature, location and magnitude. In the same way, the biological characteristics of the patient that can influence the hematoma – such as age and gender, physical activity and coagulation factors – must also be taken into account.

The physiotherapeutic treatments that can be applied to treat a hematoma can be grouped into three phases: 1) Initial phase: physical therapy aims to help the hemostasis, minimize the hematic collection and work on the inflammatory process. 2) Organisation phase: physiotherapy tries to facilitate the reabsorption of the hematoma. 3) Resolution phase: the therapeutic exercise is aimed at restoring motor skills.

The physiotherapeutic techniques and means used for the treatment of hematomas include compression and cryotherapy, as well as thermotherapy, massotherapy, electrotherapy and physical exercise with therapeutic purposes.

However, several aspects must be considered in the application of certain physiotherapeutic techniques for the treatment of hematomas in the hemophilic patient, as well as in the design of physical exercise programs for functional recovery. The intensity of the exercises and the level of impact received by joints can be of vital importance.

Chapter II - Central nervous system (CNS) is one of the most vascularized system in the human body. Despite being only about 2-3% of body-weight, it receives about 20% of the cardiac output. Although, blood flowing inside the vessels is the absolute necessity for a proper functioning, any blood leak, howsoever insignificant, creates serious clinical consequences. Hypertension remains the commonest cause of bleeding in the CNS. The clinical features of hemorrhage in the CNS are largely determined by the location, size and rapidity of the leakage. Intracerebral hemorrhage is more common than spinal hematoma, bleeding in the parenchyma being more common than in the subdural and extradural spaces. Parenchymal hemorrhage may extend into the ventricles, causing secondary complications like hydrocephalus. Subarachnoid hemorrhage is a serious event that often affects younger people. However, significant advances in the diagnostic and therapeutic approach have taken place in recent years that might improve the prognosis of this dreaded disease. Compared to the intracerebral bleeding, hemorrhages in the spinal cord are less common. Trauma, vascular malformations and anti-thrombotic drugs are the commonest caused of spinal hematoma. Owing to the constraints of space, spinal hematomas might present with rapidly developing myelopathy and constitute a neurologic urgency. Early diagnosis and appropriate interventions are usually rewarding in preventing severe long-term disabilities. In this chapter we will discuss various types of cerebro-spinal hematomas, their etiologies, clinical presentation and possible management options.

Chapter III - The infected hematomas are clinical slightly frequent entities or that in rare occasions have been communicated in the literature and therefore with an unknown morbidity-mortality. Probably some infected hematomas have been communicated in the shape of abscesses in different locations. The clinical expression of the entity is diverse and his diagnosis can turn out to be difficult. The diagnostic image technologies and the samples for the microbiological studies allow the diagnosis and precocious beginning of the treatment and the reduction of the morbidity-mortality. On having done a review of the bibliography (bibliometric search realized essentially in the MEDLINE database, using PubMed search interface), they find isolated cases and few series with scanty patients with infected hematomas. The bacteria isolated with major frequency have been *Escherichia coli*, different kinds of anaerobic, *Staphylococcus aureus*, *Salmonella sp, Mycoplasma hominis* and *Streptococcus pneumoniae*. The infected cranial hematomas have been more frequently described followed by those of abdominal location.

Chapter IV - Pelvic hematomas are collections of blood located in the pelvic peritoneal space, as a result of bleeding lacerations after operative deliveries or during gynecologic surgery. In the pelvic abdominal cavity, hematomas may take place in the uterovesical space, rectouterine pouch (Douglas space) or in paravesical, parametrial, paracervical, paravaginal or pararectal areas.

Concerning its etiology, it could be classified in obstetrical, gynecological and others causes. The most frequent obstetrical cause are puerperal hematomas that occur in 1:300 to 1:1500 deliveries and they are a potentially life-threatening complication of childbirth. The most common locations are the vulva, vaginal/paravaginal area and retroperitoneum due to an injury of uterine artery, and most rarely of the hypogastric artery during hysterotomy.

Regarding gynecological causes, surgical procedures may lead to the injury of paracervical and paravaginal vessels, ovarian vessels, uterine artery or rarely external or internal iliac vessels with major blood loss.

Other causes of pelvic hematoma include trauma, anticoagulating drugs and coagulation disease, ruptured ectopic pregnancy and ruptured of an aneurysm in the abdominopelvic vasculature.

Symptoms usually develop in the first 24 hours after delivery or surgery and vary depending on the location of the hematoma. Commonly they are associated with pain and effects caused by the hypovolemia. The three primary approaches for managing pelvic hematomas are: conservative management with observation, surgical intervention and selective arterial embolization. Evaluation of a patient with suspected postoperative or puerperal bleeding includes physical examination and assessment of vital signs and urine output. Patients who are conservatively managed should be observed closely. Surgical intervention must be carried out if growing hematoma is evidenced on physical examination or imaging studies, or hematocrite value decrease is observed.

Chapter V - An intracranial hematoma is a collection of blood in the head. The etiology is often traumatic, but can also occur in non-traumatic conditions as in the case of coagulopathy, metabolic diseases, vascular anomalies, or as a result of rupture of previously asymptomatic intracranial cysts. Depending the location, intracranial hematomas present with different symptoms and require different management, so it is important to recognize the symptoms to reach a diagnosis and to treatment as soon as possible.

Chapter VI - We wish to describe an acute case of the formation of an uncommonly large hematoma in the retroperitoneal following a vaginal intervention. This is a case report of a 72 year-old hypertensive patient on treatment with enoxaparin, among other medication, for several days before being admitted to hospital. She undergoes surgery for a cystorectocele with vaginal vault prolapse, using the vaginal way. After 36 hours she presents intense low back pain with deteriorated general state of health. The C.T. scan reveals a large hematoma approximately 16 centimeters in size with active bleeding in abdominal cavity. The case is presented for discussion and we review any medical literature concerning the appearance of this complication following gynecological interventions in patients treated with enoxparin In spite of its low prevalence following gynecological surgeries, a retroperitoneal hematoma may turn into an extremely serious complication. For this reason, the likelihood of a similar situation occurring is to be kept in mind in certain circumstances. The literature concerning the afore-mentioned complication in gynecological vaginal interventions is scarce with only rare publications of individual cases. Nevertheless, in these past years a certain number of cases related to retroperitoneal hematoma occurring spontaneously in patients being treated with enoxoparin have been published. The patients affected are fundamentally elderly, with heart disease and relative deterioration of their renal function. We were unable to discover the statistical frequency of this complication following vaginal surgery, however it is believed to be rather uncommon. In any case we consider it of interest that other specialists be aware of the possibility of its occurrence considering the seriousness of the situation.

Chapter VII - Retropharyngeal hematoma is an uncommon entity of disease of pharynx. A variety of causes are known including direct neck trauma, whiplash injury, foreign body ingestion, deep neck infection, metastatic carcinoma, anticoagulant drugs, coughing, sneezing, straining, or even spontaneous bleeding. Diagnosis can often be inferred from history but exploration may be required for confirmation. Due to pharyngeal wall swelling, it wound cause sore throat, dysphonia, dysphagia or even dyspnea while airway compromise. Physical examination may reveal stridor. In some severe cases, subcutaneous bruising over neck and anterior chest may be found. Narrowing of the pharynx can be detected simply by neck soft tissue lateral view X-ray or by endoscopic examination. Computed tomography (CT) scan or Magnetic Resonance Imaging (MRI) examination should also be necessary because the hematoma may involve inferiorly to the mediastinum causing anterior displacement of trachea or esophagus which complicate management strategy. Securing the airway is the most crucial. In traumatic cases, cervical spine immobilization is also important. Surgical evacuation of a retropharyngeal hematoma can be necessary when the hematoma is large, breathing inadequate or conservative management unsuccessful. Specific management against the possible specific cause should also be taken.

In: Hematomas: Types, Treatments … ISBN: 978-1-61942-385-5
Editors: M.F.G.Salazar…pp. 1-39

Chapter I

Haematomas, Physiotherapy and Haemophilia

J. C. Benítez-Martínez[1], *F. Querol-Fuentes*[2], *S. Pérez-Alenda*[3], *J. Casaña-Granell*[4], *and Y. Alakhdar-Mohamara*[5*]

[1]Department of Physical Therapy. University of Valencia, Spain
[2]Department of Physical Therapy. University of Valencia. University Hospital La Fe, Thrombosis and Haemostasis Unit, Haematology Service, Valencia, Spain
[3]Department of Physical Therapy. University of Valencia. University Hospital La Fe, Thrombosis and Haemostasis Unit, Haematology Service, Valencia, Spain
[4]Department of Physical Therapy. University of Valencia Spain
[5]Department of Physical Therapy. University of Valencia Spain

Abstract

Physiotherapy is a health care science steadily evolving in its fundaments as well as in its methodology. The way to tackle the treatment of hematomas has been significantly improved, even if it essentially follows the same basic principles. In the same way, the

* C/ Gascó Oliag Nº 3 46010- Valencia–Spain.

physiotherapy and physical exercise prescribed for patients with hemophilia, must take into account several transcendent aspects.

In order to develop an efficient and specific physiotherapy, the first aspect to be taken into account is the identification and knowledge of the problem, in this case, the hematomas. The second aspect will be to establish an order of priorities and objectives, which will lead the chronology of the therapeutic actions, the effects of which must also be considered.

Hematomas can be classified according to their nature, location and magnitude. In the same way, the biological characteristics of the patient that can influence the hematoma – such as age and gender, physical activity and coagulation factors – must also be taken into account.

The physiotherapeutic treatments that can be applied to treat a hematoma can be grouped into three phases: 1) Initial phase: physical therapy aims to help the hemostasis, minimize the hematic collection and work on the inflammatory process. 2) Organisation phase: physiotherapy tries to facilitate the reabsorption of the hematoma. 3) Resolution phase: the therapeutic exercise is aimed at restoring motor skills.

The physiotherapeutic techniques and means used for the treatment of hematomas include compression and cryotherapy, as well as thermotherapy, massotherapy, electrotherapy and physical exercise with therapeutic purposes.

However, several aspects must be considered in the application of certain physiotherapeutic techniques for the treatment of hematomas in the hemophilic patient, as well as in the design of physical exercise programs for functional recovery. The intensity of the exercises and the level of impact received by joints can be of vital importance.

1. Introduction

1.1. Hemophilia: General Concepts

Hemophilia is a hemorrhagic disorder; its most important and frequent manifestations affect the musculoskeletal system and it is therefore described as *hematological-based orthopedic disease requiring rehabilitation and physiotherapy*. It is a congenital disease, hereditary with recessive character, chromosome X-linked, that is, women transmit and men develop the disorder. Hemorrhages occur as a result of a quantitative and/or qualitative deficiency of coagulation factors, VIII in the case of hemophilia A, and IX in the case of hemophilia B [1]. Lack of coagulation can be life-threatening, and this mainly happens in severe hemophilia (Table 1), although traumatisms or surgery can also turn out to be fatal in mild hemophilia [2].

In the hemophilic patient the musculoskeletal bleedings prevail, being the hemarthrosis, hematomas and synovitis the most frequent musculoskeletal damages in hemophilia A and B [3, 4]. These damages lead to hemophilic arthropathy (Figure 1) at early ages, conditioning the quality of life and requiring specific hematologicalal therapy and particular physiotherapy care. The main objective of physiotherapy in hemophilia, specially in the child, is the prevention and treatment of musculoskeletal problems.

Hemophilia affects 1-2 out of 10,000 live births, although thanks to the genetic counseling a reduction in the incidence of congenital hemophilia has been achieved, at least in western countries. These figures are not yet reflected in the European statistics as a consequence of the phenomenon of immigration and the spontaneous cases (*i.e. de novo* mutations), which keep this prevalence [5, 6].

Regarding the hematological treatment, the systematic incorporation of factor replacement therapy, especially as a prophylactic treatment (Figure 2), has improved the life expectancy, which nowadays reaches the ordinary levels. However, current records of this disorder estimate the average age at 30 years and the incidence of arthropathy at around 20%.

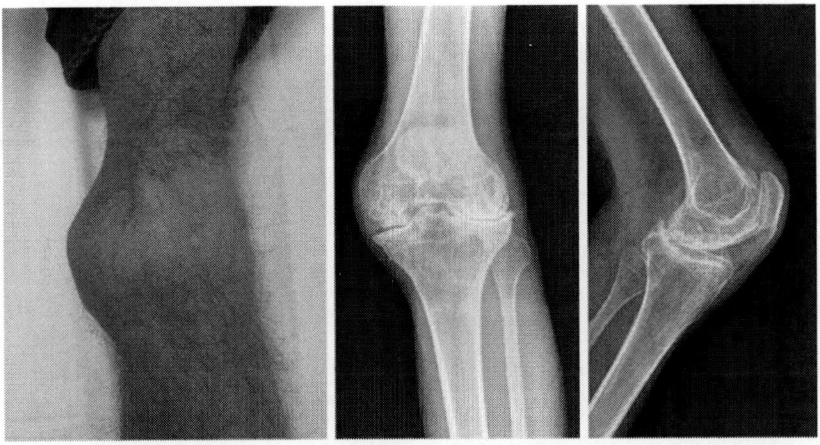

Figure 1. Severe haemophilic arthropathy in a 40 years old patient with severe haemophilia. We can see the left knee and the corresponding anteroposterior and lateral radiologic image.

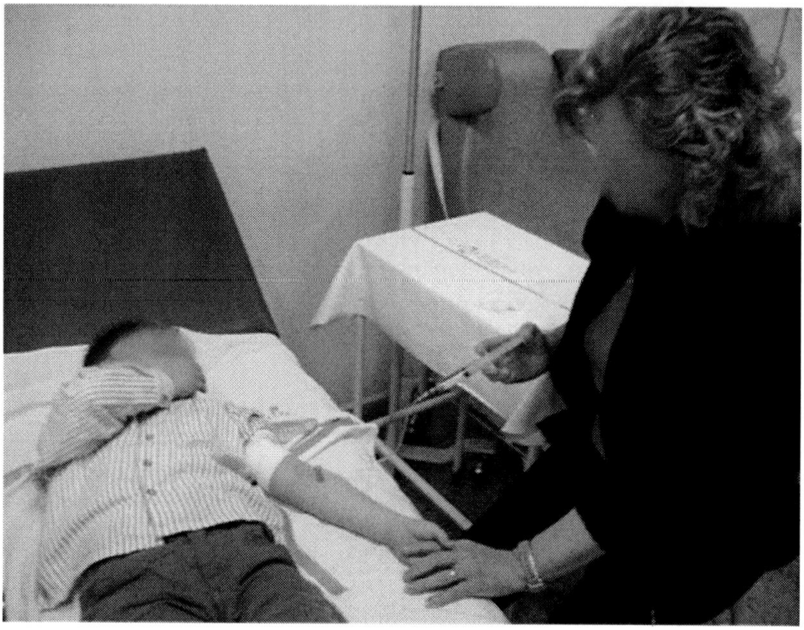

Figure 2. Intravenous infusion of factor VIII in an severe haemophilia patient.

Table 1. Classification of hemophilic clinical presentation and hemorrhagic characteristics

Classification	% factor	Hemorrhagic clinical presentation
Severe	< 1 %	Frequent hemorrhages for no apparent reason
Moderate	1-5 %	Frequent hemorrhages with minor trauma
Mild	> 5 %	Hemorrhages with serious trauma, dental procedure or surgery.
Levels higher than 40-50% don't usually suffer hemorrhages (excepting surgery or severe trauma)		

1.2. Musculoskeletal Problems in Hemophilic Patients: Hematomas

Muscular hematomas are the most frequent hemorrhagic processes after the hemarthrosis and they represent between 10% and 30% of all hemorrhages [7, 8] (Figure 3). Nevertheless, in childhood these hematomas appear at earlier ages, as children bump themselves, when crawling or trying to walk. These bleeding episodes in muscles and joints appear before the child is 2 years old in 100% of severe hemophiliacs who are not properly treated [4].

Hematomas are defined as the morbid tumefaction or swelling by blood accumulation within the tissue and can be classified into different categories: by their nature, magnitude or location. In the same way, the biological characteristics of the patient must be taken into account, *i.e.* age, gender or presence of hemophilic affection.

According to their nature, hematomas can be spontaneous and post-traumatic. A spontaneous hematoma (*i.e* without any doubt caused by a strain or unnoticed blow) requires a thorough anamnesis to find the exact cause, specially if the patient presents severe hemophilia or if it still has not been diagnosed. In the case of post-traumatic hematoma, the mechanism of injury can lead to clarify its magnitude, and therefore also the steps to take in order to stop the hemorrhage.

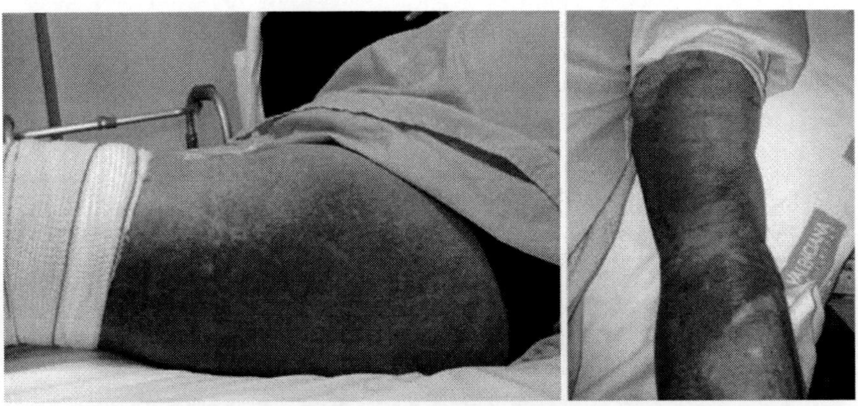

Figure 3. Haematomas with several days of evolution in adult patients with severe haemophilia. The picture on the left is a superficial hematoma in the left thigh. In the other picture we can see a hematoma, superficial and deep, in the left arm.

According to their magnitude, they can be classified into big, medium and small, which will determine the time of reabsorption. In connection with this aspect, the influence of their location is very significant, since they can threaten adjacent structures, which would be especially dangerous in the case of the nervous system.

In terms of location, they can be classified as superficial or deep. Deep hematomas can be located inside the muscle, without reaching the perimysium, or altering this structure, which causes the bleeding between the fascias. This situation makes joint/tissue mobility difficult in that area during the formation of scar tissue. Finally, according to the severity of the hematoma –depth or proximity to the bone cortical–, the hemophilic patient can develop a hemophilic pseudotumor, a serious lesion that can be mortal (Figure 4).

On the other hand, muscular hematomas can be classified as intramuscular and intermuscular. The intramuscular hematoma increases the pressure in the muscle, compressing the capillary bed. The swelling can persist and increase during the first 48 hours. Clinical presentation includes pain and tenderness to palpation, especially the first 3 days, reduced contractibility and extensibility, (*i.e.* functional deficit), and ecchymosis [9, 10]. In the case of intermuscular hematomas, the pain decreases during the first 24 hours [11].

In patients with hemophilia the muscles more frequently affected are, in this order, psoas, gastrocnemius and forearm muscles.

Therefore, the rehabilitation process of hematoma in the hemophilic patient implies 1) clinical diagnosis: hematoma location, structural damage, evaluation of risks and functional involvement and 2) therapeutic decision associated to the hematological treatment.

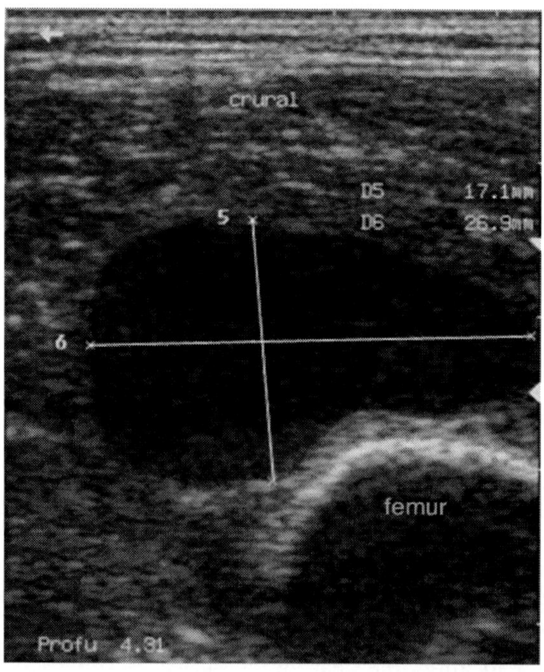

Figure 4. Ultrasound image of a hematoma in the vastus intermedius of the left leg in a child 11 years of age. The hematoma, of 26.9 x 17.1 mm, is near to the femur.

Generally speaking, rehabilitation includes the immobilization of the area affected and cryotherapy during the first 24-48 hours. The kinesiotherapy is progressive, starting with isometric exercises, being extremely careful with the muscular strain in order to prevent hemorrhage. The total load or maximal strain is authorized according to tissue healing criteria, but the control of re-bleeding with ultrasound scan is fundamental. Other physiotherapy techniques, such as magnetic therapy and ultrasound in non-thermal modality are also helpful. A muscular hematoma may encapsulate and the vascularization of this capsule will cause continuous re-bleeding. This can affect the cortical of adjacent bones, reaching them and developing the already mentioned hemophilic pseudotumor with fatal consequences (Figure 4).

1.3. Physiotherapy: Generalities for the Functional Recovery of Hematomas

Originally, physiotherapy was essentially based on massages and exercises, and the main objective of these techniques was to reduce pain and achieve functional recovery to the state prior to the injury.

Occasionally, more complex and sophisticated treatments are suggested, forgetting the essence of physiotherapy, which is the functional recovery or re-education of a function. Physical exercise offers a wide range of possibilities in that sense, allowing the improvement of different aspects of an injury, depending on the kind of exercise. Therapeutic exercise can prevent and reduce tissue rigidity, lack of stability and joint protection, muscular imbalance, incorrect performance of movements, incorrect position, and degeneration of tendons. It can also reinforce certain structures and help to integrate a correct motor sequence.

This is an outline of the steps followed to treat an injury, which presents a particular order to achieve the best progress:

1. Actions to monitor the injured structure.
2. Actions to recover the analytical function of the structure.
3. Actions to recover the global function in the motor gesture.

Physiotherapy of the *structure* implies to strive for the maximal recovery of the anatomic integrity of the tissue or tissues affected by the injury. The good knowledge of physiopathology allows suggesting therapeutic actions, which can help to improve the healing process of the damaged structure. The analytical *function* of the structure refers to the main quality for which the tissue has been conceived: contraction, stability, support or load transmission, sliding of surfaces, etc. Finally, the function in the *motor gesture* covers a global concept integrating the function of the structure and its connection to other segments, which are responsible for its integrity *(i. e.* the elements stabilizing the movement).

In physiotherapy treatment, the physical loads applied on the structure have to be strictly monitored to avoid adverse or damaging effects. Inflammation phases must be respected and the severity of the injury has to be taken into account, considering pain as an alarm of strain/stress suffered by the tissues. Here, pain and discomfort have to be differentiated. Pain can cause reflex actions like a fail or reduction in the muscular contraction, vasospasm, retraction reflex and increased tenderness/sensitization. Before the pain appears, in the active phases of mobility during the treatment, the patient can report a sensation of instability and lack of control or incapability to perform a movement. The vasospasm can be identified some hours after the exercise, for it produces an edema as a consequence of the capillary slowing-down and the consequent extravasation of plasma. This will be a parameter to assess the physical loads previously performed and adapt them to the next session of physiotherapy.

With the help of the Visual Analogue Scale (VAS) [12] pain sensitization can be monitored during the treatment session in order to evaluate how its progress. By means of direct pressure on the structure and on the most tender point of it, either with the algometer or with manual pressure, the patient is asked to mark his/her perception on the scale VAS (0 to 100mm). During the session this test can be repeated to check how the tissue endures the physical load. Increments of more than 2 points (20 mm) on the VAS would be indicative that the load is being excessive.

In terms of pain, it is important to follow the evolution immediately after the session of physiotherapy, 2-3 hours later and by the awakening next day. It is perfectly normal that after having worked on tissues which are in process of maturity, tenderness and discomfort are a little more intensive than before the exercise but, in any case, that discomfort should disappear after 2-3 hours and never produce a worsening in the ordinary physical feelings next morning. Should this occur, the physical load must be reduced in order for the tissue to be able to adapt itself to the new mechanical and functional demands and, specially, to avoid a worsening in the healing process.

2. Therapeutic Planning: Identification of the Problem

The physiotherapeutic action follows a standard sequence (Table 2).

2.1. Analysis of the Problem

In physiotherapy, apart from the diagnose (*e.g.* hematoma, location and extension), the knowledge of the mechanism in the cause of injury is also very important. This cause can be intrinsic if produced without a known external agent (*e.g.* "spontaneous" hematomas in the hemophilic patient) or extrinsic, for example caused by a direct blow or a strain. An ankle sprain by treading on an object on the floor is not the same thing as a sprain produced by a change of direction. The first case is purely traumatic but the second one can involve a possible deficit of strength, coordination, proprioception or ligament laxity, being either residual or systematic.

Table 2. Sequence in the Methodology of physiotherapy actions

		Characteristics
1	*Analysis of the Problem*	Traumatic injury, overstraining, overuse, post surgical
2	*Functión Diagnose*	Quantity (*e.g.* 1 movements of load or unload, in dialy tasks or sport activities) Quality (*e.g.* resistance, strength, ballistics, neuromuscular function, proprioception)
3	*Structure*	Bone, muscle, ligament, fascia, bursa cartilage, tendon, etc.
4	*Physiopathology*	How was the alteration caused
5	*Therapeutics*	Measures to allow/improve the healing

Injuries by overuse are more complex to treat. Formulating the hypothesis to work is more difficult since many times the identification of the damaged structures and the cause of the overuse is not easy whatsoever. Most of the reasons for these injuries lie in postural alterations, incorrect performance of a daily task and improper use of material at work or bad hygienic habits in general (*e.g.* alimentation-nutrition, rest, emotional aspect). The procedure for the treatment of post-surgical hematomas is much easier, since the information of the surgical process is completely detailed and all the limitations of the involved structures are already known.

2.2. Diagnose of the Function

Firstly, the altered function is checked to determine the possibility of movement and its characteristics, including the quantity (*i. e.* repetitions of movement in different ways: with or without load, in analytical form in a particular activity). The difficulty to perform these movements must be monitored: angular analytic movement, functional global movement, in load or unload, at the beginning of the activity or at the end, etc. All this information allows the identification of the structure and the degree of damage.

The quality is another important aspect. The possible loss of endurance must be evaluated; the capacity to perform many times a particular gesture, or the evidence of lack of strength or eccentric protection which is indicative of joint dysfunction in absence of pain. The exam of the neuromuscular function (coordination/posture) shows the injuries by overuse due to the extra work that the involved structures must perform. Finally, the proprioception is a quality not to be forgotten, since it is relevant in the prevention and recovery of injuries.

The necessary objectivity of this exam generally involves the use of standard instruments, like dynamometers, goniometers, algometers, tape measure, VAS scales and also more sophisticated ones like isokinetic evaluation, ultrasound scans, etc.

2.3. Damaged Structures

Anamnesis and clinical exploration allow a pretty exact approach to the structures affected in the tissues of the musculoskeletal system. Complementary tests (*e.g.* musculoskeletal ultrasound scans) can confirm the different structures and even detect mild injuries, which must be taken into account to monitor the progress of the healing.

2.4. Physiopathology

Some considerations must be taken into account to reflect on the physiotherapy guidelines. For example, the regeneration of the soft tissue in the locomotor system is significantly better with the application of the steady passive movement. In this way, the laxity of the ligament can be avoided. This concept is based in the fact that collagen fibers are lengthwise orientated and mechanical properties are optimized under functional loads [13]. It can be also due to the fact that the tendon tissue is more exposed to the injury or dysfunction when the postural deficit and anatomical anomalies produce alterations in the biomechanics of joints.

Chronic injuries caused by overuse are characterized by the impossibility of proper tissue healing, being the reason of this problem still unknown. The treatment of these injuries involves the early strengthening and stretching. Laboratory studies have completed the knowledge about muscular injuries and show the importance of an early mobilization [14].

When the muscle is tired, but the physical activity still has to be performed, be it in sport or at work, the tendon is selectively overused like compensatory mechanism, which finally causes the inflammation. Depending on the degree of damage or the success in the kind of treatment followed, the sub-acute phase must be reached in 3-7 days. The maturity of the collagen occurs progressively, with a moderate tension strength starting after two weeks [15].

The first physiologic mechanism to consider for the treatment of a traumatism is the evaluation of the severity of the inflammation.

Firstly, we must differentiate between acute inflammation and chronic inflammation. The latter takes place when the acute inflammation does not eliminate the agent causing the damage. The tissue is not able to come back to its normal physiological state and consequently a mechanical dysfunction appears causing a vicious circle. The tissue debility involves a repetition of the process, since there it can not resist the mechanical demands, which will cause tissue micro-breaks. The new fibers do not have time to mature and reach the correct consistence and in this way the tissue starts a process of degradation very characteristic and completely different from the acute process.

From the histological and cellular point of view, the chronic inflammation implies the replacement of leukocytes by macrophages, lymphocytes and plasmatic cells. These cells accumulate in the matrix of the floating connective tissue, highly vascularized on the area of the injury [16].

The soft musculoskeletal tissue responds to a trauma in three phases: the acute inflammatory phase (BEGINNING 0 to 7 days); proliferative phase (ORGANIZATIVE from 7 to 21 days) and the restructuring phase and maturation (RESOLUTIVE more than 21 days)

1. Acute inflammatory phase: In this phase, the ischemia, metabolic problems and damages in the cell membrane, implies the inflammation, which is characterized by the presence of cells and inflammatory markers,

exudation of fibrinogen, increment of the pressure of the capillary walls, capillary occlusion and filtration of the plasma which causes the edema in the tissue. Blood can be found in the interstice as a consequence of capillary breaking; the hematoma appears which will lead to the ecchymosis on the skin. Clinically, the inflammation appears in form of a swelling, erythema, temperature rise, pain and loss of function as a consequence of the pain and damage in the tissue, which reduces the capability to perform any particular task. The process depends on the time and it is influenced by vascular, cellular and chemical events, leading to the healing of the tissue, occasionally with formation of scars (*i. e.* adherences).

2. Proliferative phase. These changes involve a fibrin layer and a proliferation of the fibroblasts and capillaries. Inflammatory cells eliminate the fragments of damaged tissue by phagocytosis, and the fibroblasts highly and extensively increase the production of collagen (firstly collagen type 3, the weakest one, and later of collagen type 1) and other components of the extracellular matrix.
3. Maturing and restructuring phase. In this phase the content of water and proteoglycans of the healing tissue drops helping the natural viscoelastic capacity of the tissue. The fibers of collagen type I orient themselves following the lines of tension to which the tissue must respond. Approximately 6 or 8 weeks after the injury the new collagen fibers can endure a level of stress close to the ordinary level, although the final maturity of the tissue of ligaments and tendons can span from 6 to 12 months. This means that after an important injury, or an injury with long evolution, the process of healing has to be still monitored even when the symptoms subdue. Otherwise, there will be many possibilities of relapse.

In this way, the hematoma caused by a traumatism is the first step of the healing of the damaged structure but, at the same time, can become the worst complication of the traumatic event if it is not monitored and delimited, allowing fast reabsorption.

2.5. Hemostasis

As seen before, the blood extravasations produced by a traumatism, unleash a series of reactions of monitoring and damage reparation, which can be considered the first step of the healing. Thus, one of the most important aspects while monitoring the first phase of the healing is the hemostasis, which minimizes the blood extravasation.

Spontaneous or natural hemostasis can be defined as the physiologic process the fundamental function of which is to keep the blood inside the vascular system, sealing all the broken or damaged vessels.

This sealing is achieved by the formation of a solid clot which blocks the pass and depends of complex interactions among vascular wall, platelets and platelets factors, along with a complex system of physiological inhibitors and mechanisms that allow the delimitation and control of the haemostatic process.

These physiological processes can be classified in order to the better understanding of their mechanisms. There are three phases, which must be carefully chosen and applied by the physiotherapeutic techniques.

1. Vascular phase: the solution of continuity in the wall of the vessel rapidly starts the vasoconstriction, due to nervous reflexes and to substances like the serotonin, which is produced by the traumatic action itself. By closing the vessel, the loss of blood is reduced and the platelet adhesion is favored.
2. Platelet phase: the platelet thrombus is formed. The platelets continue the important mechanisms started in the first phase. Now, the function of the platelets can be classified into dynamic and plasmatic. The dynamics ones are connected to the adhesivity, aggregation, dynamics of thrombus and retractile function. The plasmatic ones liberate coagulant factors. In this phase the white thrombus is completely formed, sealing the solution of continuity. The thrombus will last 3 to 4 hours until its lysis.
3. Coagulation phase: the fibrinogen becomes an insoluble protein, the fibrin. This reaction is catabolized by the enzyme thrombin, which is not present in the plasma or in the blood circulating around. The prothrombin, its inert precursor, is the one present in the process.

The coagulant and anticoagulant action overlap in a continuous process, the objective of which is to keep the blood inside the vessels, at the same time allowing the permeability of its lumen.

As seen up to now, there will be always a hematoma associated to a traumatism, of course varying its magnitude. Logically, when one of the haemostatic mechanisms fails, the hematoma will become the most significant complication and therapeutic concern, due to the important consequences involved in its evolution and location.

3. Therapeutics

This is without any doubt the key function of the physiotherapist and will therefore be developed at length in next chapters. Now the different physiotherapeutic techniques and the importance of exercise as a therapeutic tool will be studied.

3.1. Therapeutic Approach by Objectives

"The objectives will be always the main issue even if they are the last thing achieved": once the problem, the altered function, the responsible structure, the cause of the injury and influences of the action are completely known, then it is the moment to establish priorities and plan the procedure with a clear objective. In this way, when one objective is accomplished, it will be possible to go forward.

Therapeutic objectives must be objectively measured. For example, the reduction of the edema is checked by measuring the perimeters, depending on the area, or the volume (*e.g.* introducing the affected area in a recipient with water) or by ultrasound scan, this would be the best option. The reduction of pain can be also monitored using the scale VAS, mentioned above.

The fact of knowing the physiopathology is of the uppermost importance to be able to adequate the treatment to the needs of the organism, which is itself the performer of the healing. The therapist is uniquely going to try to accelerate this process. Defining the goal and having the information about the recovery phase of the tissues will help to establish the procedure to be followed.

The objectives can be classified into three kinds:

1. General Objective: normally, the healing.
2. Specific Objectives: those applied on a particular stage of the recovery. As their name indicates, they are orientated to improve a specific aspect. There can be several and can be sequenced depending on the phases of the healing process.
3. Operative Objectives: these ones determine the tasks and techniques to be used in order to achieve a specific objective.

3.2. Physiotherapy. Phases of the Therapeutic Approach and Kinds of Therapy

In physiotherapy, the therapeutic process starts even prior to the moment when the injury occurs. This is achieved by preventive work and exercises, principally proprioception and neuromuscular assimilation. In the moment when the injury happens, the correct action of the physiotherapist is of great importance and can determinate a better and quicker recovery.

After an injury, the ideal treatment and the rehabilitation program should include four steps.

3.2.1. PRICES

Immediately after the injury, the damaged area must be treated with PRICES [17]: Protection, rest, ice, compression, elevation and stabilization (Table 3). The effect is to minimize the hemorrhage, the swelling, inflammation, cellular metabolism and pain, providing the optimal conditions for the healing. A prolonged inflammation can cause an excessive scar, which an effective treatment tries to prevent. On the other hand, the inflammation must be considered not only as an answer to the damage, but also as the first step for the healing.

3.2.2. Immobilization and Protection

The second step is the immobilization and protection of the area of the damaged tissue during the first 48 hours until the first three weeks. This will depend on the severity on the injury and it will be always relatively applied, since there are several criteria according to different researches and authors. At the early stage of the healing, the immobilization allows the invasion of fibroblasts without problems in the damaged area, which involves a proliferation of indifferent cells and production of collagen fibers. The early and intense mobilization in this period could involve the production of collagen type III and weaker tissue than the one produced during the period of optimal immobilization. On the other hand, the protection prevents secondary injuries and early distensions, as well as the increase of the length of the damaged structures of collagen. Therefore, hemostasis must be always taken into account, monitoring the first days of tissue recovery.

3.2.3. Maturation

Between five days and three weeks after the injury, the collagen and the final scar formation start [18]. In this phase, the damaged soft tissues need a monitored mobilization. Less damaged areas of the tissue and joint can be however early immobilized, sometimes even during the phase of proliferation. The prolonged immobilization must be avoided to prevent the atrophy of the cartilage, bone, muscle, tendons and ligaments [19, 20].

Monitored muscular stretching and the movement of the joints allow the orientation of the new collagen fibers parallel to the stress lines of the ordinary collagen fibers. These activities are also useful to avoid the atrophy of the tissue due to the immobilization. The treatment can be supported by other physiotherapy techniques to improve the local circulation, the proprioception, the inhibition of the pain and reinforcement of muscle-tendons units.

Table 3. Plan of the basic treatment for acute musculoskeletal injuries PRICES

P	Protection for future damages
R	Rest to avoid prolonged irritation
I	Ice to reduce the pain, hemorrhage and edema
C	Compression to support and avoid the rise of volume
E	Elevation to reduce the hemorrhage and edema
S	Support to stabilize the damaged area

3.2.4. Reincorporation

Approximately from three to eight weeks after the injury the new collagen fibers can endure a stress close to the ordinary one. The quick and total recovery of the activity is the objective of the rehabilitation. The protection will not be needed anymore, since each component of the damaged soft tissue is ready for a progressive mobilization and a rehabilitation program.

The following conclusions by different authors reveal the importance of the early mobilization and which is the way to follow in the conservative treatment.

Early Mobilization

This is the best way to avoid the contracture of the joint and its damaging consequences on the articular cartilage. The technique allows keeping and returning the proprioception of the joint. This can be transcendent in the prevention of the relapse and accelerate the total recovery. In short, Frank *et al.* [21], have suggested that the articular mobilization can help to reduce the post-injury and post-surgical pain.

Early Monitored Mobilization

Monitored clinical experiments of acute injuries of soft tissue support the results of the experimental studies and show that early monitored mobilization is better than the immobilization, not only in the primary treatment, but also in the post-surgical procedure. The superiority of this technique becomes especially clear in the periods of recuperation and return to normal activity, without risking objective or subjective results of long periods. The evidence has been systematic and convincing for many injuries: acute fracture of ankle ligaments [22, 23], after surgery for fracture of ankle ligaments [24], after surgery for chronic ankle instability [25]; injury of the ligaments of the knee [26, 27], injury of the articular cartilage [28], minimally displaced distal radius fracture [29] and complete fracture of Achilles tendon [30]. In short, the early mobilization offered very good results in many other non displaced injuries like elbow and shoulder dislocation, although not all the studies used control groups [31].

The importance of the results of this perspective must no be emphasized since they can drastically change opinions or protocols in conventional treatment. For example, in the case of patellar dislocation, two random studies carried out in Finland [32, 33] showed that after years of monitoring, the conservative treatment of acute knee-cap dislocation gave positive results, as good as the surgery followed by a similar conservative treatment.

Avoiding Atrophy

Obviously, the best method to prevent atrophy is to use the affected extremity. The complete immobilization must be minimal and often not even necessary. During the first 10 to 15 years many post-surgical protocols, especially those involving ligaments injuries in knees and ankles, have been changed, going from a complete and long immobilization to an early monitored mobilization, using elastics or other bands, devices for passive motion (CPM continuous passive motion) or a combination of them, immediately after the trauma. The active mobility or the joint and the distribution of weight are allowed for longer time and the training during the immobilization has been increased and becomes more effective [14]. Even modern treatments for fractures have considerably reduced the degree and length of immobilization [34].

Pain Control

The efficiency of an early mobilization in the prevention of the atrophy by the immobilization depends on the control over the pain, the inflammation and the growth of the edema. Inflammation and pain can cause a voluntary muscular inhibition around the affected joint. Spencer *et al.* [35] affirm that pain is not only caused by the muscular inhibition. The rise of the volume (*i. e.* edema) by itself is enough to cause it, which is also known as reflex inhibition. Therefore, the primary treatment should consist in monitoring the three factors using the early mobility in combination with other modalities of treatment like cold, analgesics, anti-inflammatory and Transcutaneous Electrical Nerve Stimulation (TENS).

Program of Re-Education

Rehabilitations programs must be tailored for each joint and kind of injury, taking into account the injured structures, which should not be submitted to an intensive mobilization. The undamaged structures should be mobilized the earlier the better. To prevent muscular dysfunctions, when immobilization is required, diverse stimuli are needed during all the process; these stimuli include strengthening, power and resistance exercises. The modern operational principle in the treatment of acute injuries in the soft tissue and during the immobilization can be defined as "within pain limits, any recurs which is not strictly forbidden, can therefore be used" [15]. This obviously requires good cooperation between the patient and the doctor or the physiotherapist who follows the case.

4. Physiotherapy in Hematomas

4.1. Instrumental and Manual Physiotherapy

4.1.1. Cryotherapy

Diverse effects can be achieved depending on the methodology applied, which will be adapted to the objective and in the phase of evolution of the hematoma:

1. Stop, slow and reduce the edema and/or hematoma: short applications of not longer than 10 minutes during the first 24/48 of the injury and compression of the injured area can cause hemostasis.

2. The reduction of the metabolism by cooling of tissues: This is interesting in the areas with poor vascularization due to edema, vasospasm and vascular compression in order to reduce the demand of oxygen in the tissue. Application times will be longer than 15 minutes, depending on the depth on the injury. In the gastrocnemius muscle, approximately after 20 minutes of application, the temperature drops 5°C [36] and it takes about 30 minutes to reach 3 cm of depth [37].
3. Reduction of the pain when slowing the nervous transmission. Applications longer than 15 minutes. Cryokinesis can be very helpful when the pain prevents the muscular movement from improving due to the existence of adherences.

The use of compression dressings can be very helpful in the application of cryotherapy, placing it over an *"ice pack"*, since this improves the cooling of superficial and deep tissues achieved by simply cooling [38]. The reduction of the temperature can be explained by the slower circulation, due to the compression [39].

4.1.2. Functional Taping

The functional taping stabilizes and protects the injured structures by combining rigid and flexible material, also allowing certain functionality of the affected segment, reducing the mechanic stress over protected structures. This taping reduces but does not completely eliminate the mechanical demands over the structure during the functional movement. This reduction will depend on the kind of dressing, the material used and the gesture performed, along with the intensity.

Many manuals show different dressing to be used in function of the structure and affected segment.

The compressive effect that must be combined with the functional taping by using foams must be taken into account in order to focus the pressure made by the dressing itself on the injured point.

4.1.3. Electro-Analgesia

Basically there are two methods: local analgesia (*e.g.* TENS, Mega current) and systematic analgesia (*e.g.* endorphin TENS or with low frequency).

Local analgesia, once applied, can last while the current is being used and no longer than some minutes after. In the same way, the analgesic effect must be felt in some minutes; otherwise it would mean that the application is not working properly due to the incorrect position of the electrodes, the type of current chosen or simply because the electro-analgesic process is not effective.

One of the most used techniques of the local analgesia is the TENS or transcutaneous electric nerves stimulation. The transmitted impulse, in transcutaneous form, stimulate the A fibers, myelinated, which transmit ascendant proprioceptive information. These fibers are sensitive to the biphasic and monophasic fibers interrupted like the ones used by the analgesia TENS. The base of the TENS effect is the theory of "gate control" postulated by Melzack and Wall [40]. The overstimulation of the A type fibers blocks the stimulus of entrance of C type fibers in the gate of posterior arc of the spinal cord, in the gelatinous substance and transmission cells (T cells) [41]. Its efficiency has been studied to reduce the pain in post-surgical patients, being significant indeed when compared to a control group and to a placebo [42], as well as in back pain [43], tensional cephalea [44] or gonarthrosis [45, 46]. A frequency between 100 and 150 Hz is normally used, along with an impulse from 150 to 250μs. The difficulty of its correct application, which must stimulate the proprioceptive fibers of the area affected, limits its effective use to those physiotherapists with the proper knowledge and experience.

This technique must be used in combination with other ones, depending on the therapeutic objective, for example in order to break the vicious circle of the contracture, which causes the pain and reduces the mobility, thus worsening the contracture. Once the pain is eliminated, while still applying the current, one can mobilize, stretch or increment the potency, depending on the objective. This technique can also be used to eliminate the reflex vasospasm that causes the pain and that will be improved by applying a massage on the affected area. This would be the only justifiable case for the analgesic electrotherapy to be used without being combined with other therapeutic measure.

The systematic analgesia, achieved by the segregation of endorphins, can be useful in very painful stages, tiredness or as sedative. This effect is achieved by the application of the current TENS with a frequency between 2 and 5 Hz and amplitude of the stimulus around 350μs. Since the effect is systematic, the application can be carried out in any area of the body, although the interscapular area is especially recommended. The intensity can be increased to achieve a significant muscular contraction and can be maintained during 30 minutes.

Nowadays there is not enough justification to use the electric stimulation in the reduction of the edema on soft tissues [47].

4.1.4. Massotherapy

The massage with therapeutic objectives is used to improve the cicatrisation of the soft tissues [48], reduce the stress and chronic pain [49, 50], improve the lymphatic drainage [51, 52, 53] and prevent the formation of adherences to the scar after surgery [54]. The massage could improve the healing of the tissues by raising the temperature, which is associated to an increment of the blood flow in skin and muscles [55, 56]. It can also improve the local blood flow, although the length of the effects is unknown. Gregory and Mars [57] could verify that after the massage with compressed air during 10 minutes, the capillary dilation persisted at least for 24h.

In the same way, the effect of the massage on pain is also very significant and it is achieved by a mechanism described in the use of TENS as the stimulus proprioceptive associated to the touch of the hands on the skin.

4.1.5. Deep Thermotherapy. Hyperthermia. Radiofrequency

The hyperthermia is a deep thermotherapy applied by means of a high frequency (0,5 MHz, 8 MHz and 430 MHz are the most recommended one in scientific literature). It is transmitted by direct touch on the patient skin. Depending on the device used it can also work without this mentioned touch. The depth achieved by rising the temperature, highly depends of the adipose tissue and device used. In general, the cellular metabolism increases [58], accelerating the regeneration, which also improves the lymphatic flow and vascular contribution [59]. The thermal effect produces vasodilatation [60], which is beneficial for the reabsorption of the hematoma. By rising the temperature in the deep tissue and combining it with stretching exercises these techniques allows the elongation of retracted tissues.

However, due to the vasodilatation produced, this technique should not be used until the haemostatic phase has finished.

4.1.6. Ultrasound (US)

High intensities ($2W/cm^2$) are recommended due to the effect of the denaturalization of proteins (*i.e.* fibrinolytic effect). This technique will be applied in case of fibroses and adherences, like in the case of encapsulated hematomas or those ones starting to become fibrous.

Mild intensities ($1W/cm^2$) have an effect on the proliferation of fibroblasts. In general, it will be applied to any process presenting damage in the conjunctive tissue.

This can be also combined with eccentric exercise to stimulate the collagen synthesis and improve its tensile proprieties, like in the case of the tendon.

The low absorption and, at the same time, the high US penetration can be seen in tissues with low content in water, while the absorption is higher in tissues with more content of proteins presenting [61], therefore, a better effect on them.

The thermal effects occur by rising the tissue temperature to 40-45°C during at least 5 minutes. Excessive thermal effects, with higher intensities, could damage the tissue [62]. However the non thermal effects are more important to the soft tissue than the thermal ones when ultrasound technique is applied [63].

Cavitation effects and micro-displacements, which have been studied in vitro, include the stimulation of the fibroplastic reparation and the synthesis of collagen [64], tissue reparation and bone healing. The ultrasound promotes the cellular proliferation in the fibroblasts on human skin [65].

Low intensity US ($0.5W/cm^2$) as well as Ga-As laser improve the biochemical and the biomechanical healing of the tendon. There are not significant statistically differences between the control group and the group of study. The combination of laser and US does not increase the positive effects. Both physical modalities can be satisfactorily used in the treatment of the tendon [66].

4.2. Therapeutic Exercise

The exercise, or more specifically, the kinesiotherapy in all its modalities: passive, active and resisted, are the fundamental base for the recovery of any injury. The current literature over severe injuries in the soft tissue of experimental kind expresses the preference of monitored early mobilization over the immobilization, in order to achieve an optimal recovery. For example, in the knee joint articulation, studies by Woo *et al.*, (revised by Woo and Hildebrand [67]) show that an experimentally induced tear in the medial collateral ligament in animals heals much better with monitored early mobilization than with immobilization.

Many of the experimental information over the effects of an early mobilization versus immobilization in terms of recovering the damaged or injured muscle comes from studies in Tampere and Turku, Finland, revised in Järvinen and Lehto [68]. In the gastrocnemius muscle of a rat, experimentally damaged, the fibers regeneration was very oft inhibited by a dense scar. Applying immobilization right after the injury reduces the area of the connective tissue formed inside the injured zone. The penetration of the muscular fibers in the connective tissue is prominent, but its orientation is complex and when the immobilization is prolonged the fibers are not parallel to the unharmed muscular fibers. Moreover, an immobilization longer than a week produced a significant atrophy of the damaged gastrocnemius muscle. In the same way, an immediate mobilization caused a dense scar, which interfered with the muscle regeneration.

In the case of the rats, the best results were achieved when the mobilization started after three or five days of immobilization. In the gastrocnemius the penetration of the muscular fiber in the connective immature tissue was optimal, and the orientation of the regenerated muscular fibers perfectly lined up with the non damaged muscular fibers. The strengthening and capacity to absorb energy was similar or even as good as the one displayed by the muscles, which were treated uniquely with an early immobilization.

In conclusion, in the damaged muscle the early mobilization must be carefully applied and respecting the initial phase of hemostasis.

Enwemeka *et al.* [69], found a significant strengthening in the Achilles tendon of rats after a recovery with early mobilization, in comparison with recovery with immobilization.

Thus, after the inflammatory phase, monitored stretching and strengthening, heals the tendon almost achieving the tensile properties of a normal one. However, the doubt remains about the fact that, even with an optimal therapy after the recovery, the collagen fibers in the tendon can lack in content, quality and orientation [70]. In the case of this deficiency, the risk of an inflammatory reaction, degeneration in tendon and fractures of tendons in later activities become dangerous.

On the other hand, the weakening of the muscular tissue starts before the injury becomes symptomatic and perhaps this has a considerable importance for the injury to be noticed. This weakening comes along with a loss of proprioceptive capacity.

After the healing, the injured tissue must accept the physical tensions that can have contributed to the injury, even if the nature is macro-traumatic or micro-traumatic.

Also, a classification should be carried out, in terms of physical exercises used as therapy. The exercises with quantitative objectives are the ones striving to improve muscular strengthening, cardiovascular or muscular resistance, hypertrophy and the range of motion (ROM). The achievements can be objectively classified in different ways (*e.g.* dynamometers, measure tape, goniometer, chronometer). The exercises with qualitative objectives are those ones trying to improve the capacity to perform a gesture, respecting the economy of movement and the harmonization of the segments involved.

The exercises with quantitative aims more frequently used in physiotherapy are those for strengthening and hypertrophy, the electro muscular stimulation (EMS), the eccentric exercises and those for flexibility. On the other hand, the qualitative exercises can be classified in stabilizing of tone exercises, those of proprioceptive re-education and postural consciousness or integration. In the following sections we will see in detail each one.

4.2.1. Strengthening Exercises and Hypertrophy

It has been proved that any musculoskeletal injury involves a loss of strength, which must be avoided since after a week it can reach higher levels. The strengthening program has to start as soon as the injury allows it.

On the other hand, the importance of the quantitative strength becomes also significant, since in only 3 days, 10% of the maximal strength can be lost. Even if the percentage of this loss can not be standardized, since endogenous and exogenous factors also play an important role, some authors speak about 1-6% of daily loss with tendency to stabilization. Other ones show reductions of 20% of the maximal strength after a week of inactivity, 25-30% after two weeks and more than 50% in four weeks. This figures use to be higher in people who regularly train.

Strength recovery is a parameter which in many occasions does not receive the required importance. In this sense, it must be taken into account in any healing process, since restoring the strength is vital in any clinical manifestation and also in order to avoid relapses. Part of the pain or discomfort can be occurring by this deficiency of stabilization and control of active movement.

Exercises to improve the strength can be of Closed Kinetic Chain or Open Kinetic Chain. The exercises in Closed Kinetic Chain offer more joint stability but, at the same time, there is a higher load transmission at joint level, reason why they are not recommended in presence of affected elements that cause articular sliding, that is, in chondromalacia or osteoarthritis. The opposite happens in the case of Open Kinetic Chain. In lower extremities, by the principle of specificity, Close Kinetic Chain exercises are always recommended, since most activities are carried out in this sense.

Regarding the training system to apply in case of hypertrophy, 10 series of 10 repetitions are recommended, with 75-80% of maximal load that the patient can manage [71]. However, the kind of training a patient is used to should be taken into account, otherwise this volume of repetitions could lead to the over-training in non-trained individuals. Therefore, the number of series must be adapted to the physical condition of the patient. In terms of week sessions, three is the average recommended.

4.2.2. Electro Muscular Stimulation (Ems)

The EMS allows, on one hand, collect a higher number of fibers than in a voluntary contraction and on the other hand, it also improves and integrates the contraction of a muscle with difficulties performing motor gestures.

The ratio intensity/time for rectangular stimuli should be calculated in order to adequate the parameters of the power to the characteristics of the patient and be able to carry out a proper dosimetry. In this way the amplitude of the stimulus to be used will be known (*i. e.* chronaxie) as well as the intensity to be applied at the beginning (*i. e.* double of the rheobase). The stimulation frequency depends on the kind of muscular fibers which must be stimulated. Thus, lower frequencies (*i. e.* 60-80Hz) are used to stimulate slow fibers, and higher ones (*i. e.* 90-120Hz.) for fibers with rapid contraction. In this sense, higher frequencies are prone to produce Delayed Onset Muscle Soreness (DOMS) [72]. Regarding times of contraction and rest, 4 seconds of contractions and 6 seconds of rest must be applied. The number of series and repetitions will follow the same methodology used for the work of strength.

Another important aspect is the kind of contraction to perform. If isometric contractions are used with the application of EMS, the risk of DOMS will be reduced [73], reason why the isometry should be used at the beginning of this therapy.

4.2.3. Eccentric Contraction Exercises

The training or eccentric work can be defined as one in which the load and resistance overcomes the strength that muscles perform to restrain or stop it. Generally the developed strength can reach figures of 130-150% of maximal isometric strength. However, sub-maximal loads of recovery between 20% to 80-90% of maximal isometric strength are used in therapeutics, in functional recovery. This will always depend on the tissue, the evolution and desired effect.

The beneficial effect of this kind of contraction over the regeneration and strengthening of tissues in tendons has been well demonstrated. In the same way, the eccentric contractions play a significant role in the stability of joints and in the muscular protection. In this sense the possible strength deficit must be checked, since the concentric capacity can be optimal but the eccentric completely reduced.

Even if disuse and inactivity can cause atrophy and weakness in the conjunctive tissues, like tendons and ligaments, the physical training can improve the maximal resistance to the tension and the quantity of absorbed energy [74]. In the same way, moments of co-contraction contribute to the dynamic joint stability [75].

The eccentric exercise and the functional recuperation are used with three different goals: regenerative therapy of the tendinous and myotendinous tissue, realignment and elastification of the muscular conjunctive tissue, preparation of the structure and the function and neuromuscular training of the control of movement (*e.g.* ballistic activity).

In general, when a program of eccentric exercises is set, muscular damage or DOMS has to be taken into account and that is why the procedure has to be progressively established.

The progression set in the eccentric actions must be:

1. Low load, slow and if necessary leaded.
2. Load increment.
3. Speed up.
4. Eccentric integrated in the functional gesture.
5. Inertial exercise *vs.* injury gesture.
6. Sport gesture/Plyometrics.

4.2.4. Flexibility Exercises

Therapeutically they are used to improve the capacity of movement in tissues and systems. This is an important quality to the right adaptability of the neuromotor system in case of overload or alteration.

Several factors determine their effects and indications:

1. Factors that determine the proportion of plastic and elastic stretching: Quantity and duration of applied force and tissue temperature.
2. Factors that determine the visco-elastic behavior of the conjunctive tissue: elastic deformation (*e.g.* stretching of short duration at high force, normal temperatures of the tissue, of cooler ones) and the viscous or plastic deformation (*e.g.* stretching of long duration with low force, high temperatures with cooling before reaching the tensor force).

3. Factors that determine the weakening of the tissue due to the deformation, like tensile forces and temperatures.

From the methodological point of view, flexibility exercises can be divided into:

1. Analytic: Those performed over a muscle or muscular group. They are used when the retraction, overload and contracture is concentrated on one of them. The segment is placed in a position in which the stretching can be comfortably kept from 10 to 30 seconds.
2. Active: these exercises are made by the patients, due to the action of the antagonist muscle or group of muscles towards the stretched group. The re-education has the utility to activate the antagonist muscle. In this way the antagonist one is toned, its contraction is integrated and at the same time the retracted muscle is stretched. This technique is often used in the last phases of the re-education due to its functionality.
3. Active tension: An isometric contraction is performed in stretching position. Its objective is the stretching of the elastic element in series and the relation muscle-aponeurosis-joint. They are used with less intensity in the traumatic injury and the proliferative one and with more intensity in the phase of tissue remodeling. In the micro-traumatic injury, or caused by overload, these exercises can be used from the beginning in order to elongate the retracted conjunctive tissue. The active tension is beneficial for muscular retractions in which the elastic element in series is affected, and its effect will be significant in tonic muscles. Isometric contraction times are about 5 seconds. The contraction must be intense when working on fast contraction fibers (IIa), going to the 15-30 seconds and mild isometric contraction in intermediate fibers (IIb), or 1-2 minutes and smooth contraction of tonic fiber (I).
4. Passive: These exercises are performed by the patient simply by action of gravity. They are used to reduce the muscular tone and relax the musculature. It is important to combine them with proper respiration and right frame of mind. They are commonly used at the end of a re-education session or training in order to improve the post-effort.
5. Passive assisted: These exercises are performed with the help of someone and it is aimed to reduce the muscle tone. They can be also used in a retraction or severe scar in the first phase in order to apply active tension lately. The insensitivity can be increased in order to direct them in the three axis of space in which the muscle can be stretched. These exercises

are applied from the beginning of injuries by micro-trauma and in the recovery of strains or important training.

6. Global: These exercises stretch several muscular groups at the same time and also the fascias which connect them. They try to eliminate compensatory synergies that can be caused by stretching a muscle and can be applied in a any moment of the recovery phase, excepting the inflammatory one. There are several methods based in this principle: Mezieres, Busquets, Global Postural Reeducation (RPG), Rolfing, etc.

4.2.5. Muscle Tonification-Stabilization Exercises

One of the principles of the training makes references to the specificity. Therefore, the functional re-education must be adapted to this principle when it is aimed to the tone-posture alterations or movement and joints stabilization.

The methodology must fundamentally display these slow and control actions and keep them, in order to train the muscular cell in this type of contractions. Also the nervous system is trained in the tone stimulations and in the sensorial integration of these actions.

The suggested exercises are firstly analytical and general ones *(i. e.* without representing the re-trained gesture) and later on, global and specific of the gesture re-trained.

In the same way, the contractions are of long duration, firstly isometric ones and then combining concentric contractions and slow eccentric ones, in order to progressively speed up and imitate the re-trained gesture. This gesture is actually most of the times a posture (*e.g.* sitting or standing posture, walking) and therefore, velocity in these actions is slow or even inexistent.

According to the type of muscle on which the action concentrates and from the quantitative point of view, i.e anatomic substrate, isotonic concentric work should be applied over phasic muscles with tendency to weakening and flaccidity. These ones, carried out systematically, can create sarcomeres in parallel (*i. e.* tendency to shorten the muscle) [76].

The performance of the work in intern length (*i.e.* complete contraction-incomplete stretching) will produce the following adaptations: light reduction of the contractile component and reduction of the total length of the muscle.

The performance of medium length (*i.e.* incomplete contraction-incomplete stretching) causes a significant reduction of the movement extent due to the loss of length in the contractile component.

4.2.6. Exercises of Proprioceptive Re-Education

This is one the earliest lost capacities, along with the strength, after an injury, being necessary for the correct muscle-joint performance. It brings protection to the stabilizing passive element and helps to harmonize the motor gesture.

Proprioceptive-sensory-motor re-educacion would be much correct as a term, since the receptors and performers of these elements are being used.

Lempereur (2003)[77] talks about neuro-motor re-programming. Its physiology responds to a circuit of reflexes-receptors/nervous system/performers. This circuit works by means of learning with "feed-back" and, progressively, thanks to the same memory of motor and kinaesthetic information, works by "feed-forward" (*i. e.* automatism).

For example, in the case of a sprain, the ligament structures, capsular and tendon structures, subcutaneous tissue and present receptors in these structures are stretched and damage. All this is going to alter the quantity and quality of the sensorial message with is connected to them. Therefore, if the message has been modified, the perception will be also changed, and consequently the established motor programs after the injury will be relatively inadequate.

By means of the practice and training of proprioception the central system learns to interpret the sensations received from its different receptors, among them the articular, muscular and proprioceptive receptors. In the same way, all these perceptions will be integrated in order to achieve the motor economy and postural comfort.

In some patients the proprioceptive perception was found to be too acute. Postures or gestures normal for other people were damaging and discomforting for them. In this case, the exercise tried to improve the quality of tissue (*e.g.* muscular stretching) and it also aimed to the reduction and reinterpretation of these perceptions.

In other cases, the opposite can also happen, *i.e.* the proprioceptives perceptions are poor. This aspect involves an overuse and damage of certain tissues; normally an anatomic injury will take place due to micro-trauma.

Nevertheless, in both situations the procedure is similar: the proprioceptive re-training. The only different aspect will be the instructions given to the patient: in the first case the patient is told to sit down, control and slow the perception, while in the other case the patient is encouraged to focus on the perception and concentration on information and feelings that exercises can offer. The patient presenting over-activity will be distracted, while the patient with infra-activity will be confronted with activities requiring maximal concentration.

4.2.7. Exercises of Consciousness and Integration of Gesture

The specific abilities to perform a gesture must be decomposed in order to train them in their most minimal components and to be able to integrate them in a model of coordinated movement. More than training the patients to perform several works or tasks, what patients really learn is how to learn [78].

Consciousness exercises or those of sensorial integration start in the first phases of any post-injury recovery. These exercises try to activate the sensorial receptors and the corresponding motor areas in the cortex.

The manual therapy and joint mobilizations are the first step for this consciousness or integration. In a sense, the fact of mobilizing a joint stimulates the proprioceptive receptors and cerebral cortex, preparing the system to the performance of the movement and the integration of sensations.

A more active implication is produced when the exercise performed is relatively new, due to the fact that it takes all the attention from patient and the conscious processes of the movement are already involved. That is why the physical exercise becomes so important in the post-injury recovery even of sedentary people. The performance of new motor actions allows the plasticity of the neuro-motor system and offers to the system new ways of adaptation in the problem solving motor/postural discomfort. In fact, it could be called neo-education and allows the neuromuscular system to adapt itself to the motor demands more easily and avoid the pain caused by more rigid and inadequate motor movement.

As stated, any exercise performed by the first time fulfils this motor consciousness. But when some specific aspects of the motor action ordinarily performed need to be stressed, there are two main possibilities.

The first one consist on, while performing the gesture, touching as well the body in order to improve the proprioceptive information on the area (*e.g.* touching the muscle to increase or reduce its contraction, touching the joint to adopt a particular position, touching all the segment to increment, reduce the speed or keeping the position). This kinaesthetic information is easy to understand by the individual, who is also being corrected.

The other procedure is the electro-stimulation. When a muscular group has to be contracted during a motor action, this can be achieved by muscular electro-stimulation. The muscular contraction during this gesture, even if artificially achieved, makes the sensorial perception caused by that contraction to be integrated in the motor scheme of the gesture, and this involves the modification of the orders of performance of this motor gesture.

When performing exercises with this aim, the patient is demanded maximal attention upon the area considered.

5. Considerations in the Physiotherapeutic Treatment of Hematomas in Haemofilic Patients

Two aspects must be considered in the physiotherapeutic treatment of the hematoma in the hemophilic patient: on one hand, the physiotherapeutic treatment of the musculoskeletal injury and, on the other the established procedure in the substitutive treatment of the deficient factor.

Firstly, the principle PRICES, already described, must be rigorously applied to any contusion, traumatism, or sign of hematoma development. Later on, in order to facilitate the reabsorption and elimination of the hematoma, other techniques already exposes can be also considered, always taking into account the consequences that any particular technique can have on the hemostasis.

The objectives of the physiotherapeutic treatment of muscular hematomas in hemophilic patient are: the inflammatory process, prevention of the bleeding, improvement the reabsorption of the hematoma and stopping a possible muscular atrophy and fibrosis, as well as the keeping of the contractile properties of the muscle and its motor function.

The physiotherapeutic measures will start after the first 24-48 hours of the stop the bleeding. During the second phase, the treatment will consist on the absolute rest of the muscle affected. Firstly the patient is kept in an antalgic position. Afterwards, another position will be set through isometric exercises, smooth tractions and different decubitus in order to situate the musculoskeletal structures in a more functional position, with less muscular shortening. Cutaneous tractions can be also used in the case of the psoas muscle in order to avoid the flex of the hip and intermittent postural treatment in prone decubitus. Cryotherapy can be used at the end of the treatment as analgesic measure [79, 80].

In the sub-acute phase, once the haemostatic process has been stabilized, one can start with analytical muscular stretching, exercises for resistance, tractions and passive kinesiotherapy until maximal lengths. In order to avoid a possible atrophy and muscle fibrosis, active, assisted and resisted kinesiotherapy can also be used.

The massotherapy is helpful to prevent the adherences, using superficial friction, sliding or massaging techniques. These techniques cause hyperemia, which helps the reabsorption of the hematoma. Pulsatile US is also recommended with 1 Mhz, depending on the depth, and intensities of 0,5-1

W/cm^2 . Moreover, it seems that its efficiency is higher if anti-inflammatory gels are used when applying the phonophoresis technique. The cryotherapy is recommended during all the phases of the treatment, due to its vasoconstrictor, anti-inflammatory and analgesic action. It should be used after kinesiotherapy or any other technique demanding a physical effect in the area with the muscular hematoma. Application time will vary between 5 and 20 minutes and it will depend on the kind of cryotherapy [81]. Another useful technique with analgesic aims for these patients is the *TENS* [80].

6. Conclusions

The conclusions can be exposed in 5 steps which should lead the action of the physiotherapist in the treatment of the hematoma, especially in the hemophilic patient:

1. Control of pain and inflammation.
2. Helping the scar healing process and regeneration, combining appropriate techniques to maximize the effects.
3. Recover the mechanical properties of the tissue.
4. Recover muscular strength and active joint stabilization.
5. Re-education of the gesture. Neuromuscular retraining and motor system in order to recover the lost function.

The musculoskeletal pathologies cause a notable functional incapability in the hemophilic patient. The close cooperation of all medical staff will be the most efficient way to avoid possible long-term non desired effects (*e.g.* physiotherapist, hematologist, nurses, radiologist).

The incidence of hematomas in hemophilic patients is significant enough to justify the use of the treatment with physiotherapy, even more when lower limbs present the more incidence of muscular problems and require kinesiotherapy for its recovery.

From the point of view of the physiotherapy, the hemophilic should be helped in terms of acting over the inflammation and improving the reabsorption of the hematoma, avoiding muscular fibroses and ankyloses of joints in order to restore the range of joint movement as it was prior to the injury and to avoid muscular atrophy.

In this way the patient will be given the optimal physical conditions in order to face all that little and repetitive injuries which reduce his/her life's quality, as time goes by.

In general, the combination of immobilization, cryotherapy, kinesiotherapy and orthotics has shown its efficiency in the treatment of muscular hematomas.

7. References

[1] Mannucci, P. M., Tuddenham, E. G. The hemophilias–from royal genes to gene therapy. *N Engl. J. Med.* 2001; 344: 1773-9.

[2] White, G. C. II, Rosendaal, F., Aledort, L. M., Lusher, J. M., Rothschild, C., Ingerslev, J. Factor VIII and Factor IX Subcommittee. Definitions in hemophilia. Recommendation of the scientific subcommittee on factor VIII and factor IX of the scientific and standardization committee of the International Society on Thrombosis and Haemostasis. *Thromb. Haemost.* 2001; 85: 560.

[3] Rodriguez-Merchan, E. C., Goddard, N. J., Lee, C. A., editors. *Musculoskeletal Aspects of Haemophilia.* Oxford: Blackwell Sciencie Ltd; 2000.

[4] Rodriguez-Merchan, E. C. Musculoskeletal complications of Hemophilia. *HSS J.* 2010; 6(1): 37-42.

[5] Stonebraker, J. S., Bolton-Maggs, P. H., Soucie, J. M., Walker, I., Brooker, M. A study of variations in the reported haemophilia A prevalence around the world. *Haemophilia.* 2010;16(1):20-32.

[6] Stonebraker, J. S., Bolton-Maggs, P. H., Michael Soucie, J., Walker, I., Brooker, M .A. study of variations in the reported haemophilia B prevalence around the world. *Haemophilia.* 2011. doi: 10.1111/j.1365-2516.2011.02588.x.

[7] Fernandez Palazzi, F., Hernandez, S. R., De Bosch, N. B., De Saez, A. R. Hematomas within the iliopsoas muscles in hemophilia patients: the Latin American experience. *Clin. Orthop. Relat. Res.* 1996; 328: 19-24.

[8] Rodriguez-Merchan, E. C., Goddard, N. J., Lee, C. A., editors. *Musculoskeletal Aspects of Haemophilia.* Oxford: Blackwell Sciencie Ltd; 2000.

[9] Norris, C. M. Sport injuries. *Diagnosis and management.* 2nd edition. Oxford: Butterworth-Heinemann; 2000.

[10] Renström, P. Muscle injuries. In: Ekstrand, J., Karlsson, J. and Hodson, A., editors. *Football medicine.* London: Martin Dunitz; 2003; 217-228.

[11] Klein, J. H. Muscular hematomas: Diagnosis and management. *J. Manipulative Physiol. Ther.* 1990; 13: 96-100.

[12] Sriwatanakul, K., Kelvie, W., Lasagna, L., Calimlim, J. F., Weis, O. F., Mehta, G. Studies with different types of analogue scales for measurement of pain. *Clin. Pharma. Ther.* 1983; 34 Suppl. 2: 234-9.

[13] Hefti, F., Stoll, T. M. Healing of ligaments and tendons. *Orthopade.* 1995; 24(3): 237-45.

[14] Renstrom, P. Sports traumatologytoday.A review of common current sports injury problems. *Ann. Chir. Gynaecol.* 1991; 80(2): 81-93.

[15] Hardy, M. A. The biology of scar formation. *Phys. Ther.* 1989; 69(12): 1014-24.

[16] Wahl, S. and Renstrom, P. Fibrosis in soft-tissue injuries.In: Leadbettter, W., Buckwalters, J. and Gordon, S . , editors. Sports-induced inflamation. Park Ridge III, *American Academy of Orthopaedic Surgeons*; 1990.

[17] Jozsa, L. and Kannus, P. A. Human Tendons: Anatomy, Physiology and Pathology.Champaign, Illinois: *Human Kinetics*; 1997.

[18] Montgomery, J. B., Steadman, J. R. Rehabilitation of the injured knee. *Clin. Sports Med.* 1985; 4(2): 333-43.

[19] Akeson, W. H., Amiel, D., Woo, S. L.-A. N. D. Immobility effects on synovial joints: the pathomechanics of joint contracture. *Biorheology.* 1980;17(1-2): 95-100.

[20] Ogata, K., Whiteside, L. A., Andersen, D. A. The intra-articular effect of various postoperative managements following knee ligament repair: an experimental study in dogs. *Clin. Orthop.* 1980; 150: 271-6.

[21] Frank, C., Akeson, W. H., Woo, S. L. Y., Amiel, D., Coutts, R. D. Physiology and therapeutic values of passive joint motion. *Clin. Orthop. Relat. Res.* 1984; 185: 113-25.

[22] Kannus, P., Renström, P. Treatment for acute tears of the lateral ligaments of the ankle: operation, cast, or early controlled mobilization? *J. Bone Joint Surg. Am.* 1991; 73(2): 305-12.

[23] Karlsson, J., Eriksson, B. I., Swärd, L. Early functional treatment for acute ligament injuries of the ankle joint. *Scand. J. Med. Sci. Sports.*1996; 6(6): 341-5.

[24] Zwipp, H., Tscherne, H., Hoffmann, R.,Wippermann, B. Therapy of fresh fibular ligament ruptures. *Orthopade.*1986; 15(6): 446-53.

[25] Karlsson, J., Lundin, O. R., Lind, K. Styf, J. Early mobilization versus immobilization after ankle ligament stabilization. *Scand. J. Med. Sci. Sports*. 1999; 9(5): 299-303.

[26] Häggmark, T., Eriksson, E. Cylinder or mobile cast brace after knee ligament injury: a clinical analysis and morphologic and enzymatic studies of changes in the quadriceps muscle. *Am. J. Sports Med.* 1979; 7(1): 48-56.

[27] Sandberg, R., Nilsson, B., Westlin, N. Hinged cast after knee ligament surgery.*Am. J. Sports Med.* 1987; 15(3): 270-4.

[28] Salter, R. B., Hamilton, H. W., Wedge, J. H., Tile, M., Torode, I. P., OR'Driscoll, S. W. et al. Clinical application of basic research on continuous passive motion for disorders and injuries of synovial joints: a preliminary report of a feasibility study. *J. Orthop. Res.* 1984; 1(3): 325-42.

[29] Stoffelen, D.,Broos, P. Minimally displaced distal radius fractures: do they need plaster treatment? *J. Trauma*. 1998; 44(3): 503-5.

[30] Saleh, M., Marshall, P. D., Senior, R., MacFarlane, A. The Sheffield splint for controlled early mobilization after rupture of the calcaneal tendon: a prospective, randomised comparison with plaster treatment. *J. Bone Joint Surg. Br.* 1992; 74(2): 206-9.

[31] Ross, G., McDevitt, E. R., Chronister, R., Ove, P. N. Treatment of simple elbow dislocation using an immediate motion protocol. *Am. J. Sports Med.* 1999; 27(3): 308-11.

[32] Nietosvaara, A. N. D. *Acute patellar dislocation in children and adolescents, dissertation*.University of Helsinki, Finland. 1996; 1-57.

[33] Nikku, R., Nietosvaara, A. N. D., Kallio, P. E., Aalto, K., Michelsson, J. E. Operative versus closed treatment of primary dislocation of the patella: similar 2-year results in 125 randomized patients. *Acta. Orthop. Scand.* 1997; 68(5): 419-23.

[34] Stoffelen, D. Broos, P. Minimally displaced distal radius fractures: do they need plaster treatment? *J. Trauma*. 1998; 44(3): 503-5.

[35] Spencer, J. D., Hayes, K. C., Alexander, I. J. Knee joint effusion and quadriceps inhibition in man. *Arch. Phys. Med. Rehabil.* 1984; 65(4): 171-7.

[36] Hartviksen, K. Ice therapy in spasticity. *Acta. Neurol. Scand.* 1962; 38(3): 79-84.

[37] Waylonis, G. W. Thephysiologiceffects of ice massage. *Arch. Phys. Med. Rehabil.* 1967; 48(1): 37-42.

[38] Knight, K. L. *Cryotherapy in sports injury management.* 1st edition. Illinois: Human Kinetics Publishers; 1995.

[39] Thorson, O. R., Lilja, B., Ahlgren, L., Hemdal, B., Westlin, N. Theeffect of local coldapplicationon intramuscular bloodflow at rest and after running. *Med. Sci. Sport Exerc.* 1985; 17: 710-3.

[40] Melzack, R., Wall, P. Pain mechanisms: a new theory. *Science.* 1965; 150: 971-9.

[41] Robinson, A. J., Snyder-Mackler, L. Eletrofisiologia Clínica: Eletroterapia e Teste Eletrofisiológico. 2ª ed. Porto Alegre: *Artmed;* 2002; 195-242.

[42] Tonella, R. M., Araújo, S., Silva, A. M. Transcutaneous electrical nerve stimulation in therelief of pain related to physical therapy after abdominal surgery. *Rev. Bras. Anestesiol.* 2006: 56(6): 630-42.

[43] Gadsby, J. G. Flowerdew, M. W. Transcutaneous electrical nerve stimulation and acupuncture-like transcutaneous electrical nerve stimulation for chronic low back pain. *Cochrane Database Syst Rev.* 2000; (2): CD000210.

[44] Vernon, H., McDermaid, C. S.,Hagino, C. Systematic review of randomized clinical trials of complementary alternative therapies in the treatment of tension type and cervicogenic headache. *Complementary Therapies in Medicine.*1999; 7: 142-55.

[45] Osiri, M., Welch, V., Brosseau, L., Shea, B., McGowan, J., Tugwell, P. *et al.* Transcutaneous electrical nerve stimulation for knee osteoarthritis. *Cochrane Database Syst. Rev.* 2000; (4): CD002823.

[46] Puett, D. W., Griffin, M. R. Published Trials of Non medicinal and Non invasive Therapies for Hip and Knee Osteoarthritis. *Ann. Intern. Med.* 1994; 121: 133-40.

[47] Wojtys, E. M., Carpenter, J. E., Ott, G. A. Electrical stimulation of soft tissues. *Instr Course Lect.* 1993; 42: 443-52.

[48] Smith, L. L., Keating, M. N., Holbert, D. Spratt, D. J.,McCammon, M. R., Smith, S. S. et al. Theeffects of athletic massage on delayed onset muscle soreness, creatinekinase and neutrophilcount: a preliminary report. *J. Orthop. Sports Phys. Ther.*1994; 19: 93-9.

[49] Sunshine, W. Field, T.,Quintino, O. R., Fierro, K., Kuhn, C.,Burman, I. et al. Fibromyalgia benefits from massage therapy and transcutaneous electrical stimulation. *J. Clin. Rheumatol.*1996; 2: 18-22.

[50] Field, T., Hernandez-Reif, M., Shaw, K. H., LaGreca, A.,Schanberg, S., Kuhn, C. Glucose levels decreased after giving massage therapy to children with diabetes mellitus. *Diabetes Spectryn.* 1997; 10: 23-5.

[51] Kurz, W., Kurz, R., Litmanovitch, Y. I., Romanoff, I. I., Pfeiffer, A. N. D. Sulman, F. G. Effect of manual lymph drainage massage on blood components and urinary neurohormones in chronic lymphhedema. *Angiology*.1981; 32: 119-27.

[52] Casley-Smith, J., Boris, M., Wendorf, S., Lasinski, B. Treatment of lymphedema of the arm the Casley-Smith method: a non-invasive method produces continued reduction. *Cancer*. 1998; 83: 2843-60.

[53] Fiaschi, E., Francesconi, G., Fiumicelli, S. N. A., Camici, M. Manual lymphatic drainage for chronic post-mastectomy lymphedema treatment. *Panminerva Med*.1998; 40: 48-50.

[54] Norris, C. *Sports injuries*. New York: Butterworth Heinemann; 1993; 109-11.

[55] Goats, G. C. The scientific basis of an ancient art: Part 2. Physiological and therapeutic effects. *Br. J. Sports Med*. 1994; 28: 153-6.

[56] Tiidus, P. M., Shoemaker, J. K. Effleurage massage, muscle blood flow and long-term post-exercise strength recovery. *Int. J. Sports Med*.1995; 16: 478-83.

[57] Gregory, M. A., Mars, M. Compressed air massage causes capillary dilation in untraumatised skeletal muscle: a morphometric and ultrastructural study. *Physiotherapy*. 2005; 91: 131-7.

[58] Horsman, M. R. Tissue physiology and the response to heat. *Int. J. Hyperthermia*. 2006; 22(3): 197-203.

[59] Akyürekli, D., Gerig, L. H., Raaphorst, G. P. Changes in muscle blood flow distribution during hyperthermia. *Int. J. Hyperthermia*. 1997; 13(5): 481-96.

[60] Nah, B. S., Choi, I. B., Oh, W. Y., Osborn, J. L., Song, C. W. Vascular thermal adaptation in tumors and normal tissue in rats. *Int. J. Radiat. Oncol. Biol. Phys*. 1996; 35(1): 95-101.

[61] Dyson, M. Mechanisms involved in therapeutic ultrasound. *Physiotherapy*. 1987; 73: 116-20.

[62] Prentice, W. E. *Therapeutic modalities in sports medicine*. 3rd edition. St Louis: Mosby; 1994.

[63] Dyson, M., Suckling, J. Stimulation of tissue repair by ultrasound: a survey of the mechanisms involved. *Physiotherapy*.1978; 64: 105-8.

[64] Webster, D. F., Harvey, W., Dyson, M., Pond, J. B. The role of ultrasound induced cavitation in the in vitro stimulation of collagen synthesis in human fibroblast. *Ultrasonics*. 1980; 18: 33-7.

[65] Zhou, S.,Schmelz, A.,Seufferlein, T., Li, A. N. D., Zhao, J., Bachem, M. G. Molecular mechanisms of low intensity pulsed ultrasound in human skin fibroblasts. *J. Biol. Chem.* 2004; 279(52): 54463-9.

[66] Demir, H., Menku, P., Kirnap, M., Calis, M., Ikizceli, I. Comparison of the effects of laser, ultrasound, and combined laser + ultrasound treatments in experimental tendon healing. *Lasers Surg. Med.* 2004; 35(1): 84-9.

[67] Woo, S. L.-A. N. D., Hildebrand, K. A. Healing of ligament injuries: from basic science to clinical practice. *Clin. Orthop.* 1997; 2(1): 63-79.

[68] Järvinen, M. J., Lehto, M. U. The effects of early mobilization and immobilization on the healing process following muscle injuries. *Sports Med.* 1993; 15(2): 78-89.

[69] Enwemeka, C. S.,Spielholz, N. I., Nelson, A. J. The effect of early functional activities on experimentally tenotomized Achilles tendons in rats. *Am. J. Phys. Med Rehabil.* 1988; 67(6): 264-9.

[70] Kannus, P., Jozsa, L., Renström, P. et al.: The effects of training, immobilization and remobilization on musculoskeletal tissue. 2: remobilization and prevention of immobilization atrophy. *Scand. J. Med. Sci. Sports.*1992; 2(4): 164-76.

[71] Cometti, G. *Les methods modernes de musculation.* Tome 1. Dijon: Universite de Bourgogne; 1989.

[72] Black, C. D., McCully, K. K. Force per active area and muscle injury during electrically stimulated contractions. *Med. Sci. Sports Exerc.* 2008; 40: 1605-15.

[73] Nosaka, K., Aldayel, A., Jubeau, M., Chen, T. C. Muscle damage induced by electrical stimulation. *Eur. J. Appl. Physiol.* 2011. DOI 10.1007/s00421-011-2086-x.

[74] Stone, M. H. Implications for connective tissue and bone alterations resulting from resistance exercise training. *Med. Sci. Sports Exerc.*1988; 20: 5162-8.

[75] Lestienne, F. Effects of inertial load and velocity on the braking process of voluntary limb movements. *Exp. Brain Res.* 1979; 35: 407.

[76] Cos Morera, M. A., Cos Morera, F. Interpretación de las alteraciones del sistema músculo esquelético. Beneficios del trabajo excéntrico and concéntrico. Efectos de la inactividad and de la inmovilización en el músculo. *Arch. Medicina del deporte.*1999; 16(74): 633-8.

[77] Lempereur, J. J. Rééducation dite "propioceptive" appliquée au rachis cervical traumatique. *Kinesithérapie Scientifique.*2003; 439; 21-7.

[78] Rothstein, J. Concentric and eccentric muscle contractions: clinical and biological perspectives. *American Physical Therapy Annual Meeting*; 1989.

[79] Querol, F., Haya, S., Aznar, J. A. Lesiones musculoesqueléticas en hemofilia: hematomas musculares. *Rev. Iberoamer. Tromb Hemostasia.* 2001; 14(2): 111-7.

[80] Querol, F., Aznar, J. A. Técnicas fisioterápicas. En: Querol, F. (director). *Guía de rehabilitación en hemofilia*. Barcelona: Ediciones Mayo; 2001; 19-27.

[81] López-Cabarcos, C. Valoración clínica del aparato locomotor. En: Querol, F. (director). *Guía de rehabilitación en hemofilia*. Barcelona: Ediciones Mayo; 2001; 9-18.

In: Hematomas: Types, Treatments ... ISBN: 978-1-61942-385-5
Editors: M.F.G.Salazar...pp. 41-78

Chapter II

Cerebrospinal Hematoma: Types, Treatment and Health Risks

Prakash R. Paliwal and Vijay K. Sharma*
Division of Neurology, National University Hospital, Singapore

Abstract

Central nervous system (CNS) is one of the most vascularized system in the human body. Despite being only about 2-3% of body-weight, it receives about 20% of the cardiac output. Although, blood flowing inside the vessels is the absolute necessity for a proper functioning, any blood leak, howsoever insignificant, creates serious clinical consequences. Hypertension remains the commonest cause of bleeding in the CNS. The clinical features of hemorrhage in the CNS are largely determined by the location, size and rapidity of the leakage. Intracerebral hemorrhage is more common than spinal hematoma, bleeding in the parenchyma being more common than in the subdural and extradural spaces. Parenchymal hemorrhage may extend into the ventricles, causing secondary complications like hydrocephalus. Subarachnoid hemorrhage is a serious event that often affects younger people. However, significant advances in the diagnostic and therapeutic

* Corresponding author: Dr. Vijay K Sharma. Associate Professor, Yong Loo Lin School of Medicine, National University of Singapore; Consultant, Division of Neurology, Dept. of Medicine, National University Hospital, 5 Lower Kent Ridge Road, Singapore 119074; Tel: +65 6772 2517;n Fax: +65 6872 3566; Email: drvijay@singnet.com.sg

approach have taken place in recent years that might improve the prognosis of this dreaded disease. Compared to the intracerebral bleeding, hemorrhages in the spinal cord are less common. Trauma, vascular malformations and anti-thrombotic drugs are the commonest caused of spinal hematoma. Owing to the constraints of space, spinal hematomas might present with rapidly developing myelopathy and constitute a neurologic urgency. Early diagnosis and appropriate interventions are usually rewarding in preventing severe long-term disabilities. In this chapter we will discuss various types of cerebro-spinal hematomas, their etiologies, clinical presentation and possible management options.

Keywords: Cerebral hemorrhage; subarachnoid hemorrhage; brain imaging.

Intracranial hemorrhage (ICH) accounts for 10% to 15% of total stroke cases and is often associated with poor outcome. It has 30 days mortality of 35-52% and half of deaths occur in first 2 days. Bleeding inside the cranial vault may occur at various places and seen more frequently than spinal hematoma. Among the intracranial hemorrhages of various kinds, bleeding within the brain parenchyma is seen more commonly than in the subdural and extradural spaces. Subarachnoid hemorrhage (SAH) constitutes one of the more serious varieties of intracranial hematomas. Although, bleeding can occur primarily into the cerebral ventricles, blood from other intracranial spaces may sometimes extend into the ventricles. Various intracranial hematomas are often associated with their respective specific predisposing factors. Accordingly, hypertension (HTN) remains the commonest etiology for parenchymal hemorrhage, occurring mainly due to the degenerative changes in arteries. Although, the usual sites for hypertensive hematoma are the deep nuclei, it may involve any other area in the cerebral hemispheres. On the other hand, subdural (SDH) and extradural hematoma (EDH) are usually related to head trauma. SDH may occur spontaneously in elderly and alcoholics. Although, head trauma may cause SAH, imaging studies are routinely performed for excluding intracranial aneurysm and arterio-venous malformations (AVM). Approach towards management often varies according to the types of ICH.

Hemorrhage in the spinal cord is less common as compared to ICH. Trauma, spinal AVM and antithrombotic agents are the commonest causes of spinal hematoma. Bleeding can occur into the epidural and subdural space and the hematoma may expand rapidly and present with progressive myelopathy.

Spinal hematomas may present as neurological emergency, even requiring urgent surgical decompression in some cases.

Spontaneous Parenchymal ICH

Spontaneous ICH is a major public health problem. The health burden of spontaneous hemorrhage is almost equal to traumatic ICH. [1,2] In general, it accounts for about 10% of total strokes. However, the incidence is approximately 20% in low-to-middle income countries that have higher mortality rates. [3] Spontaneous ICH is reported to be higher among Asians. [2] In China, where strokes outscore coronary heart disease in its incidence [4], the proportion of hemorrhagic stroke is relatively higher. [5,6] Some of the major risk factors for spontaneous ICH include male gender, hypertension, excessive consumption of alcohol, increasing age, smoking and diabetes mellitus. [7] ICH is associated with high mortality and morbidity rates, especially when the bleeding occurs due to rupture of an AVM. [8]

Location of ICH is known to have some relationship with its etiology. Accordingly, ICH involving the deep nuclei usually occurs due to hypertension while lobar ICH, especially in old age, is often associated with cerebral amyloid angiopathy. [9,10] The pathological changes in the brain tissue usually do not differentiate between primary and secondary ICH. [11] Hypertension-related ICH that commonly involves basal ganglia, thalamus, pons or cerebellum occurs due to rupture of arteries that have undergone moderately severe degenerative changes. [12] Arterial rupture often occurs at or near the bifurcation of small penetrating arteries originating from the major branches of the circle of Willis. [13] Established pathological changes for the rupture are breakage of elastic lamina, atrophy and fragmentation of smooth muscles, intimal dissection and granular or vesicular degeneration in the cells. [14] Severe atherosclerosis frequently accelerates the degenerative changes. These changes are believed to lead to fibrinoid necrosis of the vessel wall and development of focal aneurysms, increasing the risk of vessel wall rupture. [13] On the other hand, deposition of amyloid-β peptide is responsible for the degenerative changes in cerebral amyloid angiopathy in elderly individual. This process has been associated with genetic mutation involving amyloid precursor protein. [15,16] Diffuse white matter disease, believed to represent small vessel disease has also been implicated to increase the risk of ICH. [17]

Hypertension is considered as the single most important independent risk factor for ICH. [18,19] Untreated hypertension is associated with a higher risk of ICH, a factor considered responsible for the higher percentage of hemorrhagic strokes among Asians and African-Americans. [20] Some epidemiological studies have suggested that lower levels of cholesterol might be associated with higher risk of hemorragic strokes. [21-23] However, the mechanisms and the associations remain poorly understood.

Pathophysiology of Neuronal Injury

Brain parenchyma surrounding the hematoma is affected by edema and inflammatory cells. [24] The resultant edema caused mechanical temponade, contributing towards achieving hemostasis initiated by local activation of haemostatic pathways. [25] ICH may lead to clinical deterioration due to hemoatoma expansion, hydrocephalus or intraventricular extension. [26] Hematoma can expand during the first few hours due to growth of original hemorrhage or rebleeding, often associated with poor functional outcome. [27-29] These processes are believed to cause cerebral ischemia and subsequent secondary neuronal injury. [30-32] However, Schellinger et al demonstrated that hypoperfusion in the peri-hematoma regions is not predictive of outcome and proposed that the phenomenon of so-called '*ischemic penumbra of hyperacute ischemic stroke*' may not be applied to ICH patients. Contrary to acute ischemic stroke, there is salvageable ischemic tissue during very early phase of ICH. [33] Furthermore, it is argued that that instead of 'ischemic penumbra', ICH is associated with 'metabolic penumbra'. [34,35]

Other pathophysiological mechanism of neuronal injury is the formation of vasogenic edema. [36] Although, edema usually increases during the first 24 hours, it progresses further during the next few days. [37,38] The amount of edema during the first couple of days after ICH has the greatest impact on final functional outcome. [39] Exact mechanisms of the development and progression of edema after ICH are not fully understood. However, erythrocyte lysis and hemoglobin toxicity are believed to be the major contributors. [40] Presence of hemoglobin and its degradation products like oxyhemoglobin, deoxyhemoglobin, or methemoglobin in the brain parenchyma is harmful. Hemoglobin activates lipid peroxidation and neuronal injury [41] while oxyhemoglobin can induce apoptosis of neuronal cells. [42] Xi et al studied mechanism of edema formation after ICH and reported that the intracerebral infusion of erythrocyte-hemolysate induces marked edema even with normal cerebral blood flow. It appears that the edema formation is related to marked disruption of the blood brain barrier (BBB) due to the toxic effect of lysed erythrocytes and not primarily due to ischemia. [43] Iron is a potent catalyst of lipid peroxidation, and the lysis of erythrocytes contributes to BBB dysfunction. Thrombin formation during the clotting process contributes to increased lysis of erythrocytes, aggravating the edema further. [44,45] The role of ischemia of surrounding tissue in aggravating edema remains controversial.

Genetic Factors in ICH

Although, the pathogenesis of lobar and non lobar ICH is different, [46] history of ICH in the first-degree relatives is an independent risk factor for both entities. [47] An association between apoE4 genotype and cerebral amyloid angiopathy [48] has been reported with lobar ICH. [49] Recurrent lobar ICH is a feature of cerebral amyloid angiopathy, and apoE2, on top of apoE4genotype, has been implicated to increase the risk further. [50] Biffi et al, in a meta-analysis of studies related to the genetic contributions in ICH, found an association between e2 and e4 genotypes in lobar ICH predominantly associated with CAA-related ICH. They also found an association between e4 APOE and deep ICH, although a genome-wide significance was not established. [51]

Clinical Features and Diagnosis

Classically, ICH presents with neurological dysfunction of sudden onset, often with altered level of consciousness at presentation. Nausea, vomiting and headache are relatively common at onset. Neurological deficits are determined largely by the site of hemorrahge. As mentioned earlier, common sites for hypertensive hemorrhage are the putamen, thalamus, pons and cerebellum. ICH involving the putamen can present with contralateral hemiparesis, sensory loss, conjugate gaze paresis or apraxia. Thalamic bleeding can manifest with contralateral sensory disturbances, hemiparesis, gaze paresis, homonymous hemianopia, miosis, aphasia or even confusion and drowsiness. Cerebellar hematoma can cause ipsilateral ataxia and speech disturbances. Larger hematomas may cause decrease in the level of consciousness due to brainstem compression. The common presentations of bleeding in the pons can cause decreased sensorium, quadriparesis and gaze palsy. Decreased level of consciousness at presentation is common [52] that may deteriorate further during first few days [53], due to early hematoma expansion or late worsening of edema. [54] Several predictors of disease severity and early death include increasing age, initial score on the Glasgow coma scale, hematoma volume, ventricular extension and rapid enlargement of the hematoma volume. [55]

Seizures can occur at the onset of ICH and may serve as clinical marker of poor prognosis. [56,57] Seizures may be focal or generalized and usually brief in the setting of ICH. Vespa et al reported that convulsive and non convulsive status are more commonly associated with ICH as compared to ischemic stroke (27% versus 6%) [58] Seizures are more common with lobar hemorrahge and often associated with worsening of the level of consciousness, midline shift and poor outcome. Cortical EEG can reliably demonstrate the electric correlates of these seizures. [58]

Neuroimaging of ICH

Although, computed tomography (CT) is the first line investigation for ICH with good sensitivity, MRI with gradient-echo imaging has equal sensitivity to detect hyperacute ICH and is more accurate to detect microbleeds. [59] Hematoma size has been considered to be one of the most important predictors of 30-day mortality in ICH. [60] Hematoma expansion in the early phase is highly predictive of neurological deterioration [61] and an independent predictor of mortality and functional outcomes. [62] CT angiography (CTA) is a rapid and noninvasive investigation in ICH that may detect potentially treatable conditions such as aneurysms [63-67] and other vascular lesions. [68,69] Furthermore, Ryan et al demonstrated that foci of contrast enhancement may help in predicting expanding hematomas in about 91% patients. [70] Nearly half of the detected foci showed evidence of increased contrast puddling on the CT immediately after CTA.

CT scan depicts hemorrhage as a hyperdense area and multifocal hemorrhages in the brain favor traumatic etiology. CT scan can reliably estimate hematoma volume [71] as well as the severity of edema and presence of midline shift, if any. MRI gradient-echo imaging can detect ICH with equal sensitivity. T1 and T2 MRI sequences are not very sensitive but signal changes that evolve due to degradation of hemoglobin [72] in these sequences can help in determining the age of ICH. MRI can also help to detect microbleeds, whose location can guide the etiology of ICH. Accordingly, microbleeds restricted to multiple lobes may indicate amyloid angiopathy while hemorrhages in deeper areas are more likely to be due to hypertension. Multimodal MRI can also also help in characterizing the presumed perihematomal edema [73] since vasogenic edema increases the apparent diffusion coefficient (ADC) values while cytotoxic edema decreases ADC on diffusion-weighted imaging. Perfusion-weighted imaging (PWI) can help in further delineation of the critically hypoperfused regions. [74] Some of the causes of ICH such as aneurysm, arteriovenous malformations (AVM) and vasculitis may also be detected on formal digital subtraction angiography (DSA). Appearances of various types of ICH on non-contrast CT scan are shown in figure 1.

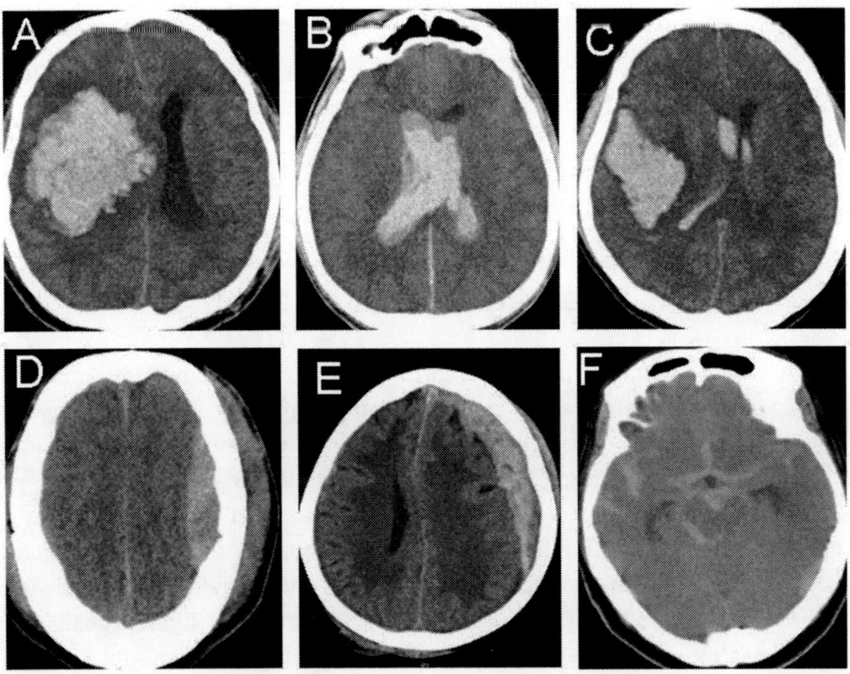

Figure 1. Appearance of various types of cerebral hemorrhages on computerized tomography. Acute hemorrhage in a hypertensive patient involving right basal ganglia region (A). Note the associated mass effect. Panel B shows primary intraventricular hemorrhage. Right parencymal hemorrhage with intraventricular extension is seen in panel C. The appearance of acute epidural hemorrhage is shown in panel D. Note the associated scalp hematoma due to head trauma. Subdural hemorrhage in a patient after a fall (E). Appearance of acute subarachnoid hemorrhage in a patient (F) due to rupture of anterior cerebral artery aneurysm.

Prevention of ICH

ICH is a neurologic emergency associated with early, and often, progressive clinical deterioration with severe deficits and high mortality. Therefore, prompt diagnosis and management is preferred for the initial management to reduce the associated mortality. [75] Hypertension remains the single most important therapeutic target in the prevention of ICH. Untreated hypertension is associated with high (3.5) odds for ICH that can be effectively reduced to 1.4 if hypertension is treated adequately. [76]

Smoking, excessive alcohol consumption and drug abuse should be discouraged for prevention of ICH. [76] Weight reduction is often recommended for ICH prevention by lowering blood pressure. [77] The DASH diet (Dietary Approaches to Stop Hypertension) suggests more intake of fruits, vegetables, low-fat dairy products and reduced total and saturated fat to control BP. [77]

Early Assessment and Management of ICH

Airway support, blood-pressure control, anticoagulation reversal, management of intracranial pressure and neurosurgical consultation are essential ingredients of early management of ICH and preferably started in the emergency department. [78-80] Approximately 30% of patients with supratentorial ICH and almost all patients with ICH in the brainstem or cerebellum present with either decreased consciousness or bulbar dysfunction necessitating intubation. [81] Rapid clinical deterioration, coupled with transtentorial herniation, mass-effect or obstructive hydrocephalus on neuroimaging demands emergent neurosurgical evaluation for possible intraventricular catheter placement or surgical evacuation with concomitant use of hyperventilation and intravenous osmotherapy. [82-84]

Acute Haemostatic Treatment

Recombinant activated factor VII (rFVIIa) is a cloned activated form of the endogenous human factor VII which is used in patients with hemophilia. Mayer et al conducted a phase 2B trial of rFVIIa in the management of acute

ICH and reported decreased hematoma expansion and reduced mortality if this agent is started within 1 hour of ICH. [85] However, a later phase 3 study FAST (factor VII in acute hemorrahgic stroke trial) did not show any significant benefit for mortality or disability in patients treated with factor VIIa. [86] A subgroup analysis of the FAST trial [87] suggested potential benefit for patients younger than 70 years with baseline hematoma volume less than 60 mL, baseline intraventricular hemorrhage volume less than 5 mL and time from onset less than or equal to 2·5 hours. A recent metanalysis of trials for factor VIIa by Yuan et al reported that factor VIIa reduces the hematoma growth but does not improve patient survival or functional outcome after ICH. Additionally, rFVIIa increased the incidence of arterial thromboembolic events. [88] Hence, routine use of Factor VIIa is not recommended for ICH.

Management of Mass-effects and Increased Intracranial Tension

Mass-effects resulting from hematomas, peri-hematoma edematous tissue and obstructive hydrocephalus are the major causes of death during the first few days after ICH. Increased intracranial pressure (ICP) can occur after large intraparenchymal or intraventricular hemorrhage. Standard ways to reduce increased ICP are elevating the head of the bed 30 to 45 degrees, intravenous mannitol (0.25-0.5 g/kg every 4 hours), intravenous furosemide, hyperventilation with a target CO_2 level of 30-35mm Hg and external ventricular drainage of cerebrospinal fluid. [76] In refractory cases, reducing brain metabolism by barbiturates or hypothermia with sedation and paralysis may be useful. Misra et al studied effect of mannitol and did not find any benefit in mortality or disability. [89] However, higher doses in preoperative settings might help in reducing the pupillary abnormalities. [90] Therefore, only short-term use of mannitol should be considered and only under special circumstances such as transtentorial herniation or acute neurological deterioration associated with high intracranial pressure or mass-effect. Hypertonic saline has longer duration of effect than mannitol and may be considered as an alternative to mannitol. [91] Hypothermia is another therapeutic option in patients with ICH. Kollmar et al found that hypothermia prevented perilesional edema in large ICH. [92] However, it is not widely available and large studies are largely lacking.

Management of Blood Pressure in ICH

The acute hypertensive response in ICH is characterised by its high prevalence, self-limiting nature, and prognostic significance. [93] Some current trials have attempted to address the issue of control of blood pressure (BP) during the early phase of ICH. The Intensive Blood Pressure Reduction in Acute Cerebral Hemorrhage (INTERACT) trial found early intensive BP-lowering treatment as clinically feasible, well tolerated and helpful in reducing hematoma growth in ICH. [94] The ongoing INTERACT-2 trial is attempting to address this issue further. According to the current practices, a systolic blood pressure (SBP) exceeding 200 mmHg or mean arterial pressure (MAP) exceeding 150 mm Hg should be controlled aggressively. BP more than 180/130 mgHg should be reduced to maintain the cerebral perfusion pressure more than 60-80 mmHg. The anti-hypertensive medications may be used as continuous intravenous infusion or as intermittent boluses. In a recent study, ICH patients treated with intravenous infusion of calcium channel blockers within 24 h of symptom onset tolerated treatment well and had low rates of neurological deterioration and hematoma expansion. [95] The study observed that intravenous-bolus-based regimens produce more variable BP control than the infusion-based regimens.

Management of Intraventricular Hemorrhage and Hydrocephalus

Intraventricular hemorrhage (IVH) is a frequent complication of ICH. The presence of IVH in hypertension- related ICH is often associated with a poor outcome. [96] IVH frequently leads to acute hydrocephalus, requiring an extraventricular drainage (EVD). [97] However, the risk of infection may outweigh the potential benefits and therefore early removal of the EVD or replacement by a ventriculo peritoneal shunt may be helpful. [98] Intraventricular fibrinolysis in combination with EVD offers a therapeutic target for increasing the clearance of intraventricular blood, enhance CSF circulation, control elevated ICP, and ultimately improve functional outcome. [99] Intraventricular injection of urokinase has been found to improve clot dissolution and reduce mortality. [100] The Clot Lysis: Evaluating Accelerated Resolution of IVH (CLEAR-IVH) trial showed similar results. [101] Some observational studies have also shown good results with endoscopic removal of IVH. [102]

Surgical Evacuation in ICH

Surgical evacuation of the ICH appears an attractive therapeutic option since this is expected to prevent hematoma expansion, decrease mass-effects, block the release of various harmful neurotoxic degradation products from the hematoma. However, early surgical intervention in the Surgical Trial in Intracerebral Hemorrhage (STICH) trial [103] did not show any significant benefits compared with the medical treatment. Although, the applicability of this trial is limited due to the high crossover rate, similar conclusions were drawn from the meta-analysis of seven trials involving early surgical evacuation in ICH. [104] Later, a subgroup analysis of STICH trial showed some positive role of surgery in patients with hematoma in the superficial layers (not more than 1 cm deeper from cortical surface) of the brain. Results of the ongoing STICH II Trial might help in establishing the role of early surgery in superficial ICH. [105] Current studies are aiming at less invasive stereotactic and endoscopic evacuation with the use of thrombolytic drugs [106] to reduce neural damage and the risk of recurrent bleeding associated with open craniotomy. A recent randomized trial showed encouraging results with the stereotactic evacuation of putaminal hematoma when the approach was associated with lower mortality and better functional recovery. [107]

Recent guidelines by the American Stroke Association [76] advocate early surgical evacuation of the ICH for patients with cerebellar hemorrhage larger than 3 cm, especially when associated with clinical deterioration, brainstem compression or hydrocephalus. [108] Although, clinical deterioration is considered as an important criteria for surgical treatment, such an approach might be more beneficial in patients with severe fourth ventricular compression even without significant neurological deterioration. [109] Accordingly, cerebellar hemorrhage is often treated successfully with external ventricular drainage that prevents the development of obstructive hydrocephalus. [110]

Seizures in ICH

Seizures, early in ICH, are independently associated with severe neurologic deficit and poor outcome. [111] Treatment of clinical seizures in ICH patients should include intravenous medications to control seizures quickly. Benzodiazepine are often the first line drugs followed by phenytoin. [76] For patients with lobar ICH, brief administration of prophylactic antiepileptic therapy soon after ICH may reduce the risk of early seizures. [76] However, strong evidence for such an approach is lacking.

Neuroprotection and other New Treatments in ICH

NXY-059, a free-radical-trapping neuroprotectant [112], was investigated in a randomised trial of 607 patients with ICH within 6 hours of symptom onset. [113] Although, compared to the placebo, NXY-059 resulted in slightly less hematoma growth, there was no significant effect on mortality, disability or final neurological deficit scores. *N*-methyl *D*-aspartate (NMDA) is involved in excitotoxicity and considered responsible for increasing risk of edema and seizure. Therefore, NMDA-antagonists may play some beneficial role in ICH. However, observations from combined Glycine Antagonist in Neuroprotection (GAIN) International and GAIN Americas trials suggest that

NMDA antagonists are not beneficial for patients with primary ICH. [114] Another neuroprotective approach in ICH has been the use of human neural stem cells injected through the bloodstream. The method appeared to promote antiapoptotic and anti-inflammatory effects of ICH and reduced the perihematomal edema. [115]

Elevated temperature is a strong risk factor for brain damage in ischemic and hemorrhagic stroke and believed to be an independent prognostic factor in these patients. Therapeutic cooling is still being investigated in acute brain injuries for its benefits in controlling ICP as well as a possible neuroprotectant strategy. The beneficial role of aggressive reduction of the brain temperature appears more important in patients with ICH. [76]

Management of Medical Complications

Bleeding from the upper gastrointestinal tracts is seen frequently in patients with ICH. Therefore, prophylactic therapy with proton pump inhibitors or H2 blockers is recommended. [116] Another common complication seen in sicker ICH patients is deep vein thrombosis (DVT) of the legs, detected by ultrasound in upto 40% cases. [117] However, the rate of clinical DVT is not that high. A randomized study showed that intermittent pneumatic compression decreased the occurrence of asymptomatic DVT when compared with elastic stockings alone and suggested intermittent pneumatic compressions for all patients. [118] The seventh American College of Chest Physicians panel recommends that a low-dose regimen of subcutaneous heparin or low-molecular-weight heparin can be started on the second day after onset of ICH in neurologically stable patients. [119] Swallowing disturbances constitute another important condition that should be recognized early in patients with ICH. Early tracheostomy in selected patients may reduce the risk of aspiration and long-term mechanical ventilation. [120]

ICH Related to Oral Anticoagulants

A population based study reported that ICH associated with oral anticoagulant use has increased from 5% in the year 1988 to 17% in 1999. This increase is most likely related to the increasing prevalence of atrial fibrillation and higher rates of oral anticoagulation in such patients. [121] Although, the risk of ICH appears to be related to the higher levels of anticoagulation, increasing age and amyloid angiopathy are important risk factors for anticoagulant-related ICH. [122] Patients with ICH related to the anticoagulant use have higher mortality, probably due to the high rates of early as well as delayed hematoma expansion [123], especially in patients with persistently elevated international normalised ratio (INR) after hospitalization. [124]

Timely reversal of the elevated INR is critical. Pharmacologic options to reverse oral-anticoagulation are vitamin K, fresh frozen plasma, prothrombin complex concentrates and rFVIIa. [125,126] An early reversal of the elevated INR (within 2 hours of the ictus) can be achieved in 84% with prothrombin complex concentrates, 39% with fresh frozen plasma, and 0% with vitamin K. Interestingly, more patients treated with rfVIIa achieved good functional outcome as compared to those who were treated with only fresh frozen plasma. [127]

The issue of restarting anticoagulation in patients who achieve good functional outcomes after ICH remains controversial. However, the current guidelines recommend that oral anticoagulants can be restarted at 7-14 days after ICH in patients at a very high risk of subsequent thromboembolism. [76]

ICH after Systemic Thrombolysis for Ischemic Stroke

ICH is the most dreaded complication of systemic thrombolysis for acute ischemic stroke. This is a complex and heterogeneous phenomenon, which involves multiple demographic, clinical, biological and hemodynamic parameters. ICH occurs mostly in the core of the infarction, suggesting the possible role of neuronal ischemia. [128] Symptomatic ICH usually occurs within 36 hours after thrombolysis. [128] In the pivotal NINDS study, 6.4% of patients developed symptomatic ICH with deterioration of the clinical status. [129] Although, the rates of symptomatic ICH were higher (10.9%)with the intra-arterial thrombolysis (Prolyse in Acute Cerebral Thromboembolism II-the PROACT II trial), the patients included in this study suffered from more severe neurological damage as compared to those included in the NINDS trial. [130] In order to minimise the risk of thrombolysis related symptomatic ICH, careful attention must be given to the glycemic control value and a strict protocol for the control of elevated blood pressure is needed during the first 24 hours following thrombolysis. [131] Compared to the rates of ICH with thrombolysis for acute ischemic stroke, the estimated rates of ICH related to intravenous tissue plasminogen activator used for acute coronary syndromes vary from about 0.07% to 1.5%. [132]

Early disruption of the blood-brain barrier appears as a reasonable explanation for the hemorrhagic complications of thrombolytic therapy. However, this has not been proven in human brain. Reperfusion is an independent predictor of blood-brain barrier disruption. [133] No effective therapy is currently available for the management of this dreaded condition. Cryoprecipitate and platelet transfusion are used routinely for thrombolysis-related ICH. The goal of therapy is the urgent replacement of the clotting factors and platelets. [76] The role of hematoma evacuation in this patient population is unknown. [134] Neuroimaging characteristics of spinocerebral hematoma after systemic thrombolysis are shown in figure 2.

ICH in Children

Nearly half of all strokes in the pediatric population are hemorrhagic. Overall mortality from ICH in children is about 25% and significant long-term disability persists in about 42% of the survivors. Previously, intracranial vascular anomalies was considered a more common cause of Pediatric ICH. [135] However, Warren et al found that brain tumors and congenital heart disease account for a greater proportion of ICH in children. [136] Unlike for adults with ICH, no medical management guidelines are available for children with ICH. [137]

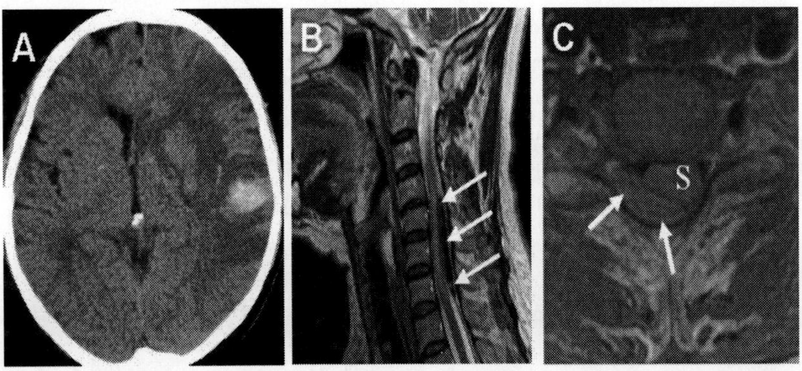

Figure 2. Spinocerebral hemorrhage after systemic thrombolysis. Computed tomographic (CT) scan showing symptomatic intracerebral hemorrhage in a patient after intravenous thrombolysis for acute left middle cerebral artery (MCA) ischemic stroke. This patient received intravenous tissue plasminogen activator (TPA) at 135minutes after symptom-onset. He showed considerable neurological recovery at 24 hours after thrombolysis. However, the brain CT showed a left MCA infarction with hemorrhagic transformation (A). Panel B and C show an acute spinal epidural hemorrhage in a patient after intravenous thrombolysis for acute brainstem stroke. This patient showed good neurological recovery during TPA infusion. However, she developed pain in the upper thoracic region and developed a new right sided weakness. MRI of the lower cervical spine showed acute epidural hemorrhage. Note the displacement of spinal cord (S) in panel c due to the hematoma. She made a good recovery at 3 months.

Subarachnoid Hemorrhage

Nontraumatic subarachnoid hemorrhage (SAH) is a neurologic emergency, characterized by extravasation of blood into the subarachnoid space. Spontaneous rupture of an intracranial aneurysm, seen in about 80% cases, is the commonest etiology of nontraumatic SAH. [138] SAH accounts for about 6-8% of all strokes and has a case fatality rate of about 40-50%. [139] The incidence of SAH has remained stable over the past 30 years. The predominant cause of death after SAH is the initial impact of the hemorrhage. [140]

The incidence increases with age [141] and relatively higher incidence is observed among females [142] and blacks. [143] Poor prognostic factors in SAH include a depressed level of consciousness on admission, age and amount of blood seen on initial CT scan. [144] The major modifiable risk factors for SAH include cigarette smoking, hypertension, cocaine use, and heavy alcohol use. [145-147] Patients with a family history of SAH among the first-degree relatives are also considered at a higher risk. [148] Some of the inherited connective tissue disorder such as polycystic kidney disease, Ehlers-Danlos syndrome (type IV), pseudoxanthoma elasticum, and fibromuscular dysplasia are also considered to be associated with SAH. [149] The risk of rupture of an intracranial aneurysm depends on its size and location, being relatively higher for anterior circulation and larger aneurysms. [150,151]

Clinical Severity and Grading of SAH

Several grading systems are used to define clinical and radiological features of SAH. The two most widely used are the Hunt and Hess grading and the World Federation of Neurological Surgeons system. [152,153] Some scoring systems grade the severity of SAH on CT scans. [154,155] Generally, higher scores predict poor prognoses for the patients. (Tables 1,2 and 3)

Clinical Features in SAH

SAH typically presents with sudden onset of severe headache, often described as thunderclap headache that is often the 'worst-headache' of the patient's life. Headache is commonly associated with nausea, vomiting, neck pain, photophobia and deterioration of the level of consciousness. [156]

Physical examination may reveal retinal hemorrhages, meningismus, diminished level of consciousness and focal neurological deficits. The focal neurological deficits can suggest the possible site of the culprit aneurysm in some cases. For example, a 3rd nerve palsy occurs commonly with the rupture of posterior communicating artery aneurysm while an anterior communication artery aneurysm rupture is expected to present with weakness of both lower extremities and abulia. Paresis of one or both lateral recti muscles of the eye balls may occur due to increased intracranial pressure and considered as a false-localizing sign in upto 50% of patients with SAH. [157]

Investigations in SAH

Head CT scan is the initial investigation of choice in patient with suspected SAH. Head CT scan can also demonstrate intraparenchymal hematomas, hydrocephalus and cerebral edema. Preferential collection of blood in a single region can help in predicting the possible site of aneurysmal rupture, especially with the rupture of aneurysms in the anterior cerebral or anterior communicating arteries. [158] Lumbar Puncture is recommended in patients with negative or equivocal CT scan. Lumbar puncture may reveal an elevated opening pressure, red blood cells and xanthochromia. Since xanthochromia take upto 12 hours to develop, some centers try to delay lumbar puncture in CT negative patients, especially with minor clinical features. The formal digital subtraction cerebral angiography remains the gold standard for detecting cerebral aneurysms. However, CT angiogram, due to its noninvasive nature and acceptable accuracy parameters is being increasingly considered as an alternative imaging modality in SAH. [159] Since small aneurysms may not be seen on the initial imaging, some patients require a repeat study after 7-14 days.

Table 1. Hunt and Hess Grading of subarachnoid hemorrhage

Grade	Characteristics
Grade 1	Asymptomatic or mild headache
Grade 2	Moderate to severe headache, nuchal rigidity, and no neurologic deficit other than possible cranial nerve palsy
Grade 3	Mild alteration in mental status (confusion, lethargy), mild focal neurologic deficit
Grade 4	Stupor and/or hemiparesis
Grade 5	Comatose and/or decerebrate rigidity

Table 2. World Federation of Neurological Surgeons Grading System for Subarachnoid Hemorrhage (WFNS) scale

Glasgow Coma Scale score	Motor deficit	Grade
15	absent	1
13-14	absent	2
13-14	present	3
7-12	Present or absent	4
3-6	Present or absent	5

Table 3. Modified Fischer scale of subarachnoid hemorrhage on computerized tomography

Grade	Subarachnoid Hemorrhage	Intraventricular Hemorrhage
0	Absent	Absent
1	Minimal	Absent in both lateral ventricles
2	Minimal	Present in both lateral ventricles
3	Thick	Absent in both lateral ventricles
4	Thick	Present in both lateral ventricles.

Treatment of SAH

Since SAH is considered an emergency, assessment of airway, breathing and circulatory hemodynamics should be performed quickly. Patient should preferably be managed in critical care unit dedicated for neurology and/or neurosurgery. [160] Main aims during the early periods of treatment for SAH are the prevention of re-bleeding and monitoring and treatment of intracranial arterial vasospasms. Blood pressure should be maintained within normal range to ensure sufficient cerebral perfusion. Analgesia should be given as required. Hyperthermia and hyperglycemia are associated with poor outcome so should be managed aggressively. [161,162] Calcium channel antagonists are known to improve the functional outcome from ischemic complications of vasospasm. Therefore, oral nimodipine is currently recommended in patients with SAH and vasospasm. [163] Although, antifibrinolytic agents are used in the early phases of SAH, their prolonged administration should be avoided to reduce the risk of cerebral ischemia and systemic thrombotic episodes. [164]

Early treatment of aneurysms has become the mainstay for preventing re-bleeding in patients with SAH. The interventions may be surgical or endovascular. However, early vascular intervention is usually preferred. [165] Endovascular treatments are relatively new [166] and sometimes may require multiple attempts to treat an aneurysm. The International Subarachnoid Aneurysm Trial (ISAT) found that the coiling of intracranial aneurysms is associated with higher rates of disability-free survival and lower risk of epilepsy. However, the re-bleeding rates are relatively higher with coiling. [167,168] In general, the best treatment for a particular patient should be decided according to the patient's age, overall medical condition, aneurysm's location and morphology in addition to its relationship to the adjacent vessels. [169] Aneurysms of vertebro-basilar system or deep in skull base are dealt with coiling whereas one with large neck diameter more suitable for clipping.

Management of Complications after SAH

Most common neurologic complications after SAH are symptomatic vasospasm followed by hydrocephalus and re-bleeding. [170,171] Re-bleeding which is more common in first 4 days increases risk of permanent disability and death. One of the most effective method of preventing re-bleeding is the vascular intervention for securing the culprit aneurysm as described previously. Symptomatic vasospasm is seen between 4-12 days and occurs due to the inflammatory reaction in arterial vessel wall. The amount of blood seen on the initial CT scan in SAH is the best predictor of subsequent vasospasm. [154,155] Transcranial Doppler (TCD) ultrasonography can be used to monitor the mean flow velocities n the major intracranial arteries. Established criteria exist for the diagnosis and grading of vasospasm in patients with SAH. [172] Vasospasm is usually treated with hypervolemia, hemodilution and induced hypertension (the so-called triple H therapy). TCD should be repeated frequently to monitor vasospasm and the effect of various treatment measures. Patients refractory to the triple-H therapy should undergo angiography followed by angioplasty or vasodilator infusion, if focal narrowing of an arterial segment is detected. Symptomatic hydrocephalus is due to decreased reabsorption of CSF due to blood and may be treated by temporary external ventricular drainage or permanent shunting. Prophylactic antiepileptics are frequently given during the initial one week as seizures can occur in 1/3rd of SAH patients and increase the risk of re-bleeding. [141]

Subdural and Extradural Hematoma

An epidural hematoma (EDH) is collection of blood between the dura mater and the skull itself while in subdural hematoma (SDH), blood accumulates between the dura mater and the arachnoid mater. EDH develops rapidly and usually due to injuries and it attains its maximum size within minutes of the initial injury, frequently associated with considerable mid-line shift. Therefore, it is considered to be an emergency in most cases. On the other hand, SDH usually develops slowly over time depending on which blood vessels are ruptured. In addition, SDH tends to spread over a larger area than an EDH as there is more space between the dura mater and the arachnoid mater than between the dura mater and skull. Thus, the amount of blood in SDH is usually much larger than EDH for causing an equal amount of pressure effects.

Extradural Hematoma

Trauma is the commonest cause of EDH. It occurs usually due to the rupture of middle meningeal vessels, dural veins or sinuses. Occasionally, EDH can occur in the absence of trauma, especially in conditions such as coagulopathies, infectious diseases of skull or vascular malformation of dura mater. Temporal lobe is the commonest site of EDH as middle meningeal artery runs very close to the inner table of skull in this region. [173] Majority of the patients show other signs of head injury. Lucid interval may be seen in 20-50% of cases of EDH. Elevation of ICP may lead to development of Cushing's reflex in some cases, presenting as markedly raised BP. However, caution should be observed in treating BP in these cases since the treatment may aggravate cerebral ischemia. [174] Skull X ray may reveal a fracture in some cases. CT scan of the brain is frequently the initial investigation of choice in which it appears as a biconvex or lenticular shaped hyperdensity on the brain's surface. The spread of EDH is limited by dura mater which is adherent to inner table of skull. The hematoma often becomes isodense in 2-4 weeks after the initial trauma and later becomes hypodense to the brain tissue. Occasionally, acute blood may appear isodense or even hypodense areas, probably due to the ongoing hemorrhage or a low hemoglobin level. [175] EDH in the posterior fossa may even be complicated by hydrocephalus.

Initial management of EDH may be conservative if it is small in size. However, the patients should be monitored for deterioration. [176,177] Patient with significantly raised intracranial pressure should be managed by osmotic agents and/or hyperventilation. Craniotomy and evacuation of the EDH with inspection of the dura is the preferred procedure in patients requiring surgery. Endovascular embolization to minimize bleeding during the acute stage and evacuation using closed suction drain are some of the novel therapeutic approaches that can be used in some patients. [178,179]

Subdural Hematoma

SDH is usually caused by trauma but it may also occur spontaneously, especially in the elderly. Anticoagulation may also contribute to it. The neuroimaging characteristics of SDH are usually determined by its size, location and the age of hematoma (acute/ subacute/ chronic). Acute SDH (seen within first 72 hours) appear as a hyperdensity over the surface of brain on the CT scan. SDH between 3 to 20 days is called as subacute and appear as isodense or hypodense to the brain surface. Chronic SDH is more than 3 weeks old and appears hypodense on the plain CT. Acute SDH is commonly associated with extensive primary brain injury. Accordingly, upto 82% of comatose patients with acute SDH demonstrate parenchymal contusions. [180] Chronic SDH is considered as a common treatable cause of dementia, and seen with brain atrophy due to old age, alcoholism and/or old stroke. In acute SDH due to head injury, tear in the bridging veins is the usual source of bleeding. Similar to any other mass lesion, SDH can result in increased intracranial pressure and cause subsequent complications. Chronic SDH may occur de novo in atrophic brain or may evolve from liquifaction of acute SDH.

Since acute SDH is usually due to head injury, it is more common in males. The clinical features depend on size of hematoma and associated parenchymal brain injury. SDH patients may present with altered sensorium, ipsilateral dilation of the pupil and contralateral weakness. Chronic SDH is more commonly seen in the elderly patients. Clinical course in chronic SDH is insidious and often presents with altered sensorium, headache, gait disturbances and cognitive decline and even mimic parkinsonism. [181] Chronic SDH is usually bilateral and may appear heterogeneous due to different age of bleeding.

Surgical evacuation via craniotomy is often considered in patients with an acute SDH thicker than 5 mm and any neurological signs such as lethargy or other change in mental status or a focal neurological deficit. Bullock et al suggested that an acute SDH with a thickness greater than 10 mm or a midline shift greater than 5 mm on CT scan should be surgically evacuated, regardless of the patient's Glasgow Coma Scale score. [182] On the other hand, for chronic SDH, surgery should be considered in symptomatic patients or associated with significant mass effect. SDH may also be drained by burr holes. Bedside drainage via twist-drill craniotomy has also been described for chronic SDH. [183] The recently introduced Subdural Evacuating Port System has also been reported to have good results. [184]

Spinal Hematoma

Hemorrhage in the spinal cord is far less common as compared to ICH. Spinal hemorrhage may occur due to trauma, arteriovenous malformation or related to anti-thrombotic agents. [185] Bleeding in the spinal cord may occur into the epidural or subdural space or within spinal cord. A rapidly expanding spinal hematoma can present with rapidly developing myelopathy and a neurologic urgency requiring surgical decompression. Arteriovenous malformations and trauma may be associated with spinal epidural hematoma (SEH) and hematomyelia. However, bleeding into the spinal subdural space is frequently seen with trauma and anticoagulation. [186] Hematomyelia is caused by bleeding within the spinal cord in which the blood tends to dissect longitudinally above and below the primary site of hemorrhage, disrupting gray matter more than white matter. Irrespective of the space, spinal hematoma presents with symptoms of painful myelopathy. It is associated with sudden severe localized back pain with weakness in the extremities, sensory loss below the level of lesion and sphincter disturbances. Spinal MRI is the preferred imaging modality for confirming the diagnosis. Spinal angiography or CT angiography may be performed to detect the cause of bleeding in some cases.

Coagulopathy should be corrected in patients when this is the underlying cause. Surgery is indicated if hematomyelia is expanding with worsening neurological symptoms or arteriovenous malformation is the underlying cause of bleeding. [187] Spinal angiomas can also be approached by catheter based techniques like coiling or embolization. Focal radiation therapy like gamma knife can also be considered for spinal arteriovenous malformations. After initial surgical treatment, rehabilitation is usually required to improve the functional status. Symptomatic medications are often required for spasticity and neuropathic pain. Loss of bladder control may be treated with anticholinergics and/or intermittent catheterization. Prognosis of spinal hematoma usually correlates with severity of initial deficit and may be improved with prompt surgical intervention in suitable cases.

In conclusion, acute spinocerebellar hematomas are catastrophic events and require prompt diagnosis. Early diagnosis and appropriate treatment is often successful in achieving complete recovery in some and limiting the long term disabilities in a significant proportion of patients.

References

[1] Lovelock CE, Molyneux AJ, Rothwell PM (2007) Change in incidence and aetiology of intracerebral haemorrhage in Oxfordshire, UK, between 1981 and 2006: a population-based study. *Lancet Neurol* 6: 487-493.

[2] Van Asch CJ, Luitse MJ, Rinkel GJ, van der Tweel I, Algra A, et al. (2010) Incidence, case fatality, and functional outcome of intracerebral haemorrhage over time, according to age, sex, and ethnic origin: a systematic review and metaanalysis. *Lancet Neurol* 9: 167-176.

[3] Feigin VL, Lawes CM, Bennett DA, Barker- Collo SL, Parag V. (2009) Worldwide stroke incidence and early case fatality reported in 56 population-based studies: a systematic review. *Lancet Neurol* 8: 355-369.

[4] Wu Z, Yao C, Zhao D, Wu G, Wang W, Liu J, Zeng Z, Wu Y. (2001). Sino-MONICA Project: a collaborative study on trends and determinants in cardiovascular diseases in China, part I: morbidity and mortality monitoring. *Circulation* 103:462-468.

[5] Zhang LF, Yang J, Hong Z, Yuan GG, Zhou BF, Zhao LC, Huang YN, Chen J, Wu YF. (2003) Proportion of different subtypes of stroke in China. *Stroke* 2091-2096.

[6] Yang QD, Niu Q, Zhou YH, Liu YH, Xu HW, Gu WP, Tian FF, Xie YQ, Zhang L, Xia J. (2004) Incidence of cerebral hemorrhage in the Changsha community. *Cerebrovasc Dis* 17:303-313.

[7] Ariesen MJ, Claus SP, Rinkel GJ, Algra A (2003) Risk factors for intracerebral hemor rhage in the general population: a systematic review. *Stroke* 34: 2060-2065.

[8] Van Beijnum J, Lovelock CE, Cordonnier C, Rothwell PM, Klijn CJ, et al. (2009) Outcome after spontaneous and arteriovenous malformation-

related intracerebral haemorrhage: population- based studies. *Brain* 132: 537-543.

[9] Ritter MA, Droste DW, Hegedus K, Szepesi R, Nabavi DG, et al. (2005) Role of cerebral amyloid angiopathy in intracerebral hemorrhage in hypertensive patients. *Neurology* 64: 1233-1237.

[10] Jackson CA, Sudlow CL. (2006) Is hypertension a more frequent risk factor for deep than for lobar supratentorial intracerebral haemorrhage? *J Neurol Neurosurg Psychiatry* 77: 1244-1252.

[11] Steiner T, Rosand J, Diringer M. (2006) Intracerebral hemorrhage associated with oral anticoagulant therapy: current practices and unresolved questions. *Stroke* 37:256-262.

[12] Qureshi AI, Tuhrim S, Broderick JP, Batjer HH, Hondo H. Hanley DF. (2001) Spontaneous intracerebral hemorrhage, *N Engl J Med* 344:1450-1460.

[13] Takebayashi S, Kaneko M. (1983) Electron microscopic studies of ruptured arteries in hypertensive intracerebral hemorrhage. *Stroke* 14: 28-36.

[14] Mizutani T, Kojima H, Miki Y. (2000) Arterial dissections of penetrating cerebral arteries causing hypertension-induced cerebral hemorrhage. *Neurosurg* 93: 859-862.

[15] Rosand J, Hylek EM, O'Donnell HC, Greenberg SM. (2000) Warfarin associated hemorrhage and cerebral amyloid angiopathy: a genetic and pathologic study, *Neurology* 55: 947-951.

[16] Rost NS, Greenberg SM, Rosand J. (2008) The genetic architecture of intracerebral hemorrhage. *Stroke* 39: 2166-2173.

[17] Smith EE, Gurol ME, Eng JA, et al. (2004) White matter lesions, cognition, and recurrent hemorrhage in lobar intracerebral hemorrhage, *Neurology* 63:1606-1612.

[18] Woo D, Sauerbeck LR, Kissela BM, Khoury JC, Szaflarski JP, Gebel J, et al. (2002) Genetic and environmental risk factors for intracerebral hemorrhage: preliminary results of a population-based study. *Stroke* 33:1190-1196.

[19] Kissela BM, Sauerbeck L, Woo D, Khoury J, Carrozzella J, Pancioli A, et al. (2002) Subarachnoid hemorrhage: a preventable disease with a heritable component. *Stroke* 33:1321-1326.

[20] Daniel W, Mary H, Padmini S, Brett K, Jane K, Alexander S, et al. (2004) Effect of untreated hypertension on hemorrhagic dtroke. *Stroke* 35:1703-1708.

[21] Okumura K, Iseki K, Wakugami K, Kimura Y, Muratani H, Ikemiya Y, Fukiyama K. Low serum cholesterol as a risk factor for hemorrhagic stroke in men: a community-based mass screening in Okinawa, Japan. *Jpn Circ J* 63:53-58.
[22] Segal AZ, Chiu RI, Eggleston-Sexton PM, Beiser A, Greenberg SM. (1999) Low cholesterol as a risk factor for primary intracerebral hemorrhage: a casecontrol study. *Neuroepidemiology* 1999;18:185-193.
[23] Iribarren C, Jacobs DR, Sadler M, Claxton AJ, Sidney S. (1996) Low total serum cholesterol and intracerebral hemorrhagic stroke: is the association confined to elderly men? The Kaiser Permanente medical care program. *Stroke*;27:1993-1998.
[24] Qureshi AI, Suri MF, Ostrow PT et al.(2003) Apoptosis as a form of cell death in intracerebral hemorrhage. *Neurosurgery* 52: 1041-1047.
[25] Fujii Y, Takeuchi S, Harada A, Abe H, Sasaki O, Tanaka R. (2001) Hemostatic activation in spontaneous intracerebral hemorrhage. *Stroke* 32:883-890.
[26] Qureshi AI, Mendelow AD, Hanley DF (2009) Intracerebral haemorrhage. *Lancet* 373:1632-1644.
[27] Brott T, Broderick J, Kothari R, Barsan W, Tomsick T, et al. (1997) Early hemorrhage growth in patients with intracerebral hemorrhage. *Stroke* 28:1-5.
[28] Davis SM, Broderick J, Hennerici M, Brun NC, Diringer MN, et al. (2006) Hematoma growth is a determinant of mortality and poor outcome after intracerebral hemorrhage. *Neurology* 66:1175-1181.
[29] Ji N, Lu JJ, Zhao YL, Wang S, Zhao JZ (2009) Imaging and clinical prognostic indicators for early hematoma enlargement after spontaneous intracerebral hemorrhage. *Neurol Res* 31:362-366.
[30] Carhuapoma JR, Wang PY, Beauchamp NJ, Keyl PM, Hanley DF, Barker PB. (2000) Diffusion-weighted MRI and proton MR spectroscopic imaging in the study of secondary neuronal injury after intracerebral hemorrhage. *Stroke*;31:726-732.
[31] Videen TO, Dunford-Shore JE, Diringer MN, Powers WJ. (1999) Correction for partial volume effects in regional blood flow measurements adjacent to hematomas in humans with intracerebral hemorrhage: implementation and validation. *J Comput Assist Tomogr*;23:248-256.
[32] Ropper AH, Zervas NT. (1982) Cerebral blood flow after experimental basal ganglia hemorrhage. *Ann Neuro* 11:266-271.

[33] Schellinger PD, Fiebach JB, Katrin H, Kristina B, Berk O, Rainer K, et al. (2003) Stroke MRI in Intracerebral Hemorrhage :Is There a Perihemorrhagic Penumbra? *Stroke* 34:1674-1679.

[34] Zazulia AR, Diringer MN, Videen TO, Adams RE, Yundt K, et al. (2001) Hypoperfusion without ischemia surrounding acute intracerebral hemorrhage. *J Cereb Blood Flow Metab* 21:804-810.

[35] Herweh C, Juttler E, Schellinger PD, Klotz E, Jenetzky E, et al. (2007) Evidence against a perihemorrhagic penumbra provided by perfusion computed tomography. *Stroke* 38:2941-2947.

[36] Butcher KS, Baird T, MacGregor L, Desmond P, Tress B, et al. (2004) Perihematomal edema in primary intracerebral hemorrhage is plasma derived. *Stroke* 35:1879-1885.

[37] Zazulia AR, Diringer MN, Derdeyn CP, Powers WJ (1999) Progression of mass effect after intracerebral hemorrhage. *Stroke* 30: 1167-1173.

[38] Gebel JM, Jr., Jauch EC, Brott TG, Khoury J, Sauerbeck L, et al. (2002) Natural history of perihematomal edema in patients with hyperacute spontaneous intracerebral hemorrhage. *Stroke* 33:2631-2635.

[39] Gebel JM Jr, Jauch EC, Brott TG, et al. (2002) Relative edema volume is a predictor of outcome in patients with hyperacute spontaneous intracerebral hemorrhage. *Stroke* 33:2636-2641.

[40] Xi G, Keep RF, Hoff JT. (1998) Erythrocytes and delayed brain edema formation following intracerebral hemorrhage in rats. *J Neurosurg* 89:991-996.

[41] Gutteridge JM. (1987) The antioxidant activity of haptoglobin towards haemoglobin-stimulated lipid peroxidation. *Biochim Biophys Acta* 917:219-223.

[42] Ogihara K, Zubkov AY, Bernanke DH, Lewis AI, Parent AD, Zhang JH. (1999) Oxyhemoglobin-induced apoptosis in cultured endothelial cells. *J Neurosurg* 91:459-465.

[43] Xi G, Hua Y, Bhasin RR, Ennis SR, Keep RF, Hoff JT. (2001) Mechanisms of edema formation after intracerebral hemorrhage: Effects of extravasated red blood cells on blood flow and blood-brain barrier integrity. *Stroke* 32:2932-2938.

[44] Lee KR, Betz AL, Keep RF, Chenevert TL, Kim S, Hoff JT. (1995) Intracerebral infusion of thrombin as a cause of brain edema. *J Neurosurg*.;83:1045-1050.\

[45] Xi G, Wagner KR, Keep RF, Hua Y, de Courten-Myers GM, Broderick JP, Brott TG, Hoff JT. (1998) The role of blood clot formation on early

edema development following experimental intracerebral hemorrhage. *Stroke* 29:2580-2586.

[46] Sacco RL. (2000) Lobar intracerebral hemorrhage. *N Engl J Med* 342:276-279.

[47] Daniel W, Laura RS, Brett MK, Jane CK, Jerzy PS, James G, et al. (2002) Genetic and environmental risk factors for intracerebral hemorrhage : Preliminary results of a population-based study. *Stroke* 33:1190-1196.

[48] Greenberg SM, Rebeck GW, Vonsattel JP, Gomez-Isla T, Hyman BT. (1995) Apolipoprotein E epsilon 4 and cerebral hemorrhage associated with amyloid angiopathy. *Ann Neurol* 38:254-259.

[49] Greenberg S, Briggs M, Hyman B, Kokoris G, Takis C, Kanter D, Kase C, Pessin M. (1996) Apolipoprotein E4 is associated with the presence and earlier onset of hemorrhage in cerebral amyloid angiopathy. *Stroke* 27:1333-1337.

[50] O'Donnell HC, Rosand J, Knudsen KA, Furie KL, Segal ZA, Chiu RI, Ikeda D, Greenberg SM. (2000) Apolipoprotein E genotype and the risk of recurrent lobar intracerebral hemorrhage. *N Engl J Med* 342:240-245.

[51] Biffi A, Sonni A, Anderson CD, Kissela B, Jagiella JM, Schmidt H, Conde JJ, Hansen BM, et al. (2010) Variants at APOE Influence Risk of Deep and Lobar Intracerebral Hemorrhage. *Ann Neurology* 68:934-943.

[52] Moon JS, Janjua N, Ahmed S et al. (2008) Prehospital neurologic deterioration in patients with intracerebral hemorrhage. *Crit Care Med* 36:172-175.

[53] Leira R, Davalos A and Silva Y *et al.* (2004) Early neurologic deterioration in intracerebral hemorrhage: predictors and associated factors. *Neurology* 63:461467.

[54] Mayer SA, Sacco RL, Shi T, Mohr JP. (1994) Neurologic deterioration in noncomatose patients with supratentorial intracerebral hemorrhage. *Neurology* 44:1379-1384.

[55] Hemphill JC, Bonovich DC, Besmertis L, Manley GT, Johnston SC. (2001) The ICH score: a simple, reliable grading scale for intracerebral hemorrhage. *Stroke* 32:891-897.

[56] Berger AR, Lipton RB, Lesser ML, Lantos G, Portenoy RK. (1988) Early seizures following intracerebral hemorrhage: implications for therapy. Neurology 38:1363-1365.

[57] Labovitz DL, Hauser WA, Sacco RL. (2001) Prevalence and predictors of early seizure and status epilepticus after first stroke. *Neurology* 57:200-206.

[58] Vespa PM, O'Phelan K, Shah M, Mirabelli J, StarkmanS, Kidwell C, et al. (2003) Acute seizures after intracerebral hemorrhage A factor in progressive midline shift and outcome. *Neurology* 60:1441-1446.

[59] Kidwell CS, Chalela JA, Saver JL *et al.*(2004) Comparison of MRI and CT for detection of acute intracerebral hemorrhage. *JAMA* 292:1823-1830.

[60] Broderick JP, Brott TG, Duldner JE, Tomsick T, Huster G. (1993) Volume of intracerebral hemorrhage: a powerful and easy-to-use predictor of 30-day mortality. *Stroke* 24:987-993.

[61] Kazui S, Naritomi H, Yamamoto H, Sawada T, Yamaguchi T. (1996) Enlargement of spontaneous intracerebral hemorrhage: incidence and time course. *Stroke* 27:1783-1787.

[62] Davis SM, Broderick J, Hennerici M, Brun NC, Diringer MN, Mayer SA, Begtrup K, Steiner T. (2006) Recombinant Activated Factor VII Intracerebral Hemorrhage Trial Investigators. Hematoma growth is a determinant of mortality and poor outcome after intracerebral hemorrhage. *Neurology* 66:1175-1181.

[63] Matsumoto M, Sato M, Nakano M, Endo Y, Watanabe Y, Sasaki T, Suzuki K, Kodama N. (2001) Three-dimensional computerized tomography angiography guided surgery of acutely ruptured cerebral aneurysms. *J Neurosurg* 94:718-727.

[64] Villablanca JP, Jahan R, Hooshi P, Lim S, Duckwiler G, Patel A, Sayre J, Martin N, Frazee J, Bentson J, Vinuela F. (2002) Detection and characterization of very small cerebral aneurysms by using 2D and 3D helical CT angiography. *AJNR Am J Neuroradiol* 23:1187-1198.

[65] Hoh BL, Cheung AC, Rabinov JD, Pryor JC, Carter BS, Ogilvy CS. (2004) Results of a prospective protocol of computed tomographic angiography in place of catheter angiography as the only diagnostic and pretreatment planning study for cerebral aneurysms by a combined neurovascular team. *Neurosurgery* 54:1329-1340.

[66] Hope JK, Wilson JL, Thomson FJ. (1996) Three-dimensional CT angiography in the detection and characterization of intracranial berry aneurysms. *AJNR Am J Neuroradiol* 17:439-445.

[67] Korogi Y, Takahashi M, Katada K, Ogura Y, Hasuo K, Ochi M, Utsunomiya H, Abe T, Imakita S. (1999) Intracranial aneurysms: detection with three dimensional CT angiography with volume rendering: comparison with conventional angiographic and surgical findings. *Radiology* 211:497-506.

[68] Sanelli PC, Mifsud MJ, Stieg PE. (2004) Role of CT angiography in guiding management decisions of newly diagnosed and residual arteriovenous malformations. *AJR Am J Roentgenol* 183:1123-1126.

[69] Coenen VA, Dammert S, Reinges MH, Mull M, Gilsbach JM, Rohde V. (2005) Image-guided microneurosurgical management of small cerebral arteriovenous malformations: the value of navigated computed tomographic angiography. *Neuroradiology* 47:66-72.

[70] Ryan W, Richard IA, Allan J, Demetrios JS, David G, George T, Sean S. (2007) CTAngiography "Spot Sign" predicts hematoma expansion in acute intracerebral hemorrhage. *Stroke* 38:1257-1262.

[71] Zimmerman RD, Maldjian JA, Brun NC, Horvath B, Skolnick BE.(2006) Radiologic Estimation of Hematoma Volume in Intracerebral Hemorrhage Trial by CT Scan: *American Journal of Neuroradiology* 27:666-670.

[72] Atlas SW, Thulborn KR. Intracranial hemorrhage. In: *Magnetic Resonance Imaging of the Brain and Spine.* 3rd ed. Philadelphia, Pa: Lippincott Williams & Wilkins; 2002:773-832.

[73] Carhuapoma JR, Hanley DF, Banerjee M, Beauchamp NJ. (2003) Brain edema after human cerebral hemorrhage: a magnetic resonance imaging volumetric analysis. *J Neurosurg Anesthesiol* 15:230-233.

[74] Olivot JM, Mlynash M, Zaharchuk G, Straka M, Bammer R, Schwartz N Lansberg MG, et al. (2009) Perfusion MRI (Tmax and MTT) correlation with xenon CT cerebral blood flow in stroke patients. *Neurology* 72:1140-1145.

[75] Diringer MN, Edwards DF. (2001) Admission to a neurologic/neurosurgical intensive care unit is associated with reduced mortality rate after intracerebral hemorrhage. *Crit Care Med* 29:635-640.

[76] Broderick J, Connolly S, Feldmann E, et al. (2007) Guidelines for the management of spontaneous intracerebral hemorrhage in adults: 2007 update: a guidelines from the American Heart Association/American Stroke Association Stroke Council, High Blood Pressure Research Council, and the Quality of Care and Outcomes in Research Interdisciplinary Working Group. *Stroke* 38:2001- 2023.

[77] Goldstein LB, Adams R, Alberts MJ, et al. (2006) Primary prevention of ischemic stroke: a guideline from the American Heart Association/American Stroke Association Stroke Council: cosponsored by the Atherosclerotic Peripheral Vascular Disease Interdisciplinary Working Group, Cardiovascular Nursing Council, Clinical Cardiology

Council, Nutrition, Physical Activity, and Metabolism Council, and the Quality of Care and Outcomes Research Interdisciplinary Working Group. *Stroke* 37:1583-1633.

[78] Qureshi AI, Mohammad YM, Yahia AM et al.(2005) A prospective multicenter study to evaluate the feasibility and safety of aggressive antihypertensive treatment in patients with acute intracerebral hemorrhage. *J Intensive Care Med* 20:34-42.

[79] Qureshi AI, Geocadin RG, Suarez JI, Ulatowski JA. (2000) Long-term outcome after medical reversal of transtentorial herniation in patients with supratentorial mass lesions, *Crit Care Med* 28:1556-1564.

[80] Goldstein JN, Thomas SH, Frontiero V, *et al.* (2006) Timing of fresh frozen plasma administration and rapid correction of coagulopathy in warfarin-related intracerebral hemorrhage. *Stroke* 37:151-155.

[81] Gujjar AR, Deibert E, Manno EM, Duff S, Diringer MN. (1998) Mechanical ventilation for ischemic stroke and intracerebral hemorrhage: indications, timing, and outcome. *Neurology* 51: 447-451.

[82] Naff NJ, Tuhrim S. (1997) Intraventricular hemorrhage in adults: complications and treatment. *New Horizons* 5: 359-363.

[83] Naff NJ, Carhuapoma JR, Williams MA, et al. (2000) Treatment of intraventricular hemorrhage with urokinase: effects on 30-day survival. *Stroke* 31: 841-847.

[84] Naff NJ, Hanley DF, Keyl PM, *et al.* (2004) Intraventricular thrombolysis speeds blood clot resolution: results of a pilot, prospective, randomized, double-blind, controlled trial, *Neurosurgery* 54: 577-583.

[85] Mayer SA, Brun NC, Begtrup K, et al. (2005) Recombinant activated factor VII for acute intracerebral hemorrhage. *N Engl J Med* 352:777-785.

[86] Mayer SA, Brun NC, Begtrup K, et al. (2008) Efficacy and safety of recombinant activated factor VII for acute intracerebral hemorrhage. *N Engl J Med* 358:2127-2137.

[87] Dziedzic T, Szczudlik A, Klimkowicz A, Rog TM, Slowik A.(2003) Is mannitol safe for patients with intracerebral hemorrhages? Renal considerations. *Clin Neurol Neurosurg* 105: 87-89.

[88] Yuan ZH, Jiang JK, Huang WD, Pan J, Zhu JY, Wang JZ. (2010) A meta analysis of the efficacy and safety of recombinant activated factor VII for patients with acute intracerebral hemorrhage without hemophilia. *J Clin Neurosci* 17:685-93.

[89] Misra UK, Kalita J, Ranjan P, Mandal SK. (2005) Mannitol in intracerebral hemorrhage: a randomized controlled study. *J Neurol Sci* 234: 41-45.

[90] Cruz J, Minoja G, Okuchi K. (2002) Major clinical and physiological benefits of early high doses of mannitol for intraparenchymal temporal lobe hemorrhages with abnormal pupillary widening: a randomized trial. *Neurosurgery* 51:628-637.

[91] Suarez JI , Qureshi AI , Bhardwaj A , et al.(1998) Treatment of refractory intracranial hypertension with 23.4% saline. *Crit Care Med* 26:1118-1122.

[92] Kollmar R, Staykov D, Do¨rfler A, Schellinger P, Schwab S, Bardutzky J. (2010) Hypothermia Reduces Perihemorrhagic Edema After Intracerebral Hemorrhage. *Stroke* 41:1684-1689.

[93] Qureshi AI. (2008) Acute hypertensive response in patients with stroke: pathophysiology and management. *Circulation* 118:176-187.

[94] Anderson CS, Huang Y, Wang JG, Arima H, Neal B, Peng B, Heely E, et al. (2008) Acute Hypertensive response in intracerebral haemorrhage: is treatment safe and helpful?. *The Lancet Neurology* 7: 374-375.

[95] Qureshi AI, Mohammad YM, Yahia AM *et al.* (2005) A prospective multicenter study to evaluate the feasibility and safety of aggressive antihypertensive treatment in patients with acute intracerebral hemorrhage. *J Intensive Care Med* 20: 34-42.

[96] Ohwaki K, Yano E, Nagashima H, Hirata M, Nakagomi T, Tamura A. (2006) Surgery for patients with severe supratentorial intracerebral hemorrhage. *Neurocrit Care* 5:15-20.

[97] Hanley DF. (2009) Intraventricular hemorrhage and ICH outcomes: severity factor and treatment target. *Stroke* 40:1533-1538.

[98] Yilmazlar S, Abas F, Korfali E. (2005) Comparison of ventricular drainage in poor grade patients after intracranial hemorrhage. *Neurol Res* 27:653-656.

[99] Demaerschalk BM. (2008) Fibrinolytic therapy for intraventricular hemorrhage: is the answer becoming clear yet? *Eur J Neurol* 15:320-322.

[100] Vespa P, McArthur D, Miller C, et al. (2005) Frameless stereotactic aspiration and thrombolysis of deep intracerebral hemorrhage is associated with reduction of hemorrhage volume and neurological improvement. *Neurocrit Care* 2:274- 281.

[101] Nyquist P, Hanley DF. (2007) The use of intraventricular thrombolytics in intraventricular hemorrhage. *J Neurol Sci* 261:84-88.

[102] Longatti PL, Martinuzzi A, Fiorindi A, Maistrello L, Carteri A. (2004) Neuroendoscopic management of intraventricular hemorrhage, *Stroke* 35: e35-38.

[103] Mendelow AD, Gregson BA, Fernandes HM *et al.* (2005) Early surgery versus initial conservative treatment in patients with spontaneous supratentorial intracerebral haematomas in the International Surgical Trial in Intracerebral Haemorrhage (STICH): a randomised trial. *Lancet* 365:387-397.

[104] Fernandes HM, Gregson B, Siddique S, Mendelow AD. (2000) Surgery in intracerebral hemorrhage. The uncertainty continues. *Stroke* 31:2511-2516.

[105] STICH II Trial. http://www.ncl.ac.uk/stich/

[106] JP Broderick. (2005) The STICH trial: what does it tell us and where do we go from here? *Stroke* 36:1619-1620.

[107] Hattori N, Katayama Y, Maya Y, Gatherer A. (2004) Impact of stereotactic hematoma evacuation on activities of daily living during the chronic period following spontaneous putaminal hemorrhage: a randomized study. *J Neurosurg* 101:417-420.

[108] Morioka J, Fujii M, Kato S, et al. (2006) Surgery for spontaneous intracerebral hemorrhage has greater remedial value than conservative therapy. *Surg Neurol* 65:67-72.

[109] Lyden PD, Shuaib A, Lees KR, et al.(2007) Safety and tolerability of NXY059 for acute intracerebral hemorrhage: the CHANT Trial. *Stroke* 38:2262-2269.

[110] Yamamoto T, Nakao Y, Mori K, Maeda M. (2006) Endoscopic hematoma evacuation for hypertensive cerebellar hemorrhage. *Minim Invasive Neurosurg* 49:173-178.

[111] Claassen J, Mayer SA, Kowalski RG, Emerson RG, Hirsch LJ. (2004) Detection of electrographic seizures with continuous EEG monitoring in critically ill patients. *Neurology* 62:1743-1748.

[112] St Louis EK, Wijdicks EF, Li H. (1998) Predicting neurologic deterioration in patients with cerebellar hematomas. *Neurology* 51:1364-1369.

[113] Sumer MM, Acikgoz B, Akpinar G. (2002) External ventricular drainage for acute obstructive hydrocephalus developing following spontaneous intracerebral haemorrhages, *Neurol Sci* 23:29-33.

[114] Haley EC, Thompson JLP, Levin B, Davis S, Lees KR, Pittman JG et al. (2005) Gavestinel does not improve outcome after acute intracerebral

hemorrhage: An analysis from the GAIN International and GAIN Americas studies. *Stroke* 36:1006-1010.

[115] Pluchino S, Martino G. (2008) Neural stem cell-mediated immunomodulation: repairing the haemorrhagic brain. *Brain* 131:604-605.

[116] Misra UK, Kalita J, Pandey S, Mandal SK, Srivastava M. (2005) A randomized placebo controlled trial of ranitidine versus sucralfate in patients with spontaneous intracerebral hemorrhage for prevention of gastric hemorrhage. *J Neurol Sci* 239:5-10.

[117] Ogata T, Yasaka M, Wakugawa Y, Inoue T, Ibayashi T, Okada Y. (2008) Deep venous thrombosis after acute intracerebral hemorrhage. *J Neurol Sci* 272: 83-86.

[118] Lacut K, Bressollette L, Le Gal G *et al.*(2005) Prevention of venous thrombosis in patients with acute intracerebral hemorrhage. *Neurology* 65:865- 869.

[119] Albers GW, Amarenco P, Easton JD, Sacco RL, Teal P. (2004) Antithrombotic and thrombolytic therapy for ischemic stroke: the seventh ACCP Conference on Antithrombotic and Thrombolytic Therapy. *Chest* 126:483S–512S.

[120] Huttner HB, Kohrmann M, Berger C, Georgiadis D, Schwab S. (2006) Predictive factors for tracheostomy in neurocritical care patients with spontaneous supratentorial hemorrhage. *Cerebrovasc Dis* 21:159-165.

[121] Flaherty ML, Kissela B, Woo D *et al.*(2007) The increasing incidence of anticoagulant-associated intracerebral hemorrhage. *Neurology* 68:116-121.

[122] Rosand J, Hylek EM, O'Donnell HC, Greenberg SM.(2000) Warfarin-associated hemorrhage and cerebral amyloid angiopathy: a genetic and pathologic study. *Neurology* 55: 947-951.

[123] Flibotte JJ, Hagan N, O'Donnell J, Greenberg SM, Rosand J. Warfarin, hematoma expansion, and outcome of intracerebral hemorrhage. *Neurology* 63:1059-1064.

[124] Huttner HB, Schellinger PD, Hartmann M, *et al.* (2006) Hematoma growth and outcome in treated neurocritical care patients with intracerebral hemorrhage related to oral anticoagulant therapy: comparison of acute treatment strategies using vitamin K, fresh frozen plasma, and prothrombin complex concentrates. *Stroke* 37:1465-1470.

[125] Goldstein JN, Thomas SH, Frontiero V *et al.* (2006) Timing of fresh frozen plasma administration and rapid correction of coagulopathy in warfarin-related intracerebral hemorrhage. *Stroke* 37:151-155.

[126] Brody DL, Aiyagari V, Shackleford AM, Diringer MN. (2005) Use of recombinant factor VIIa in patients with warfarin-associated intracranial hemorrhage. *Neurocrit Care* 2:263-267.

[127] Roitberg B, Emechebe-Kennedy O, Amin-Hanjani S, Mucksavage J, Tesoro E. (2005) Human recombinant factor VII for emergency reversal of coagulopathy in neurosurgical patients: a retrospective comparative study. *Neurosurgery* 57:832-836.

[128] The National Institute of Neurological Disorders and Stroke rt-PA Stroke Study Group. (1997) Intracerebral hemorrhage after intravenous t-PA therapy for ischemic stroke. *Stroke* 28:2109-2118.

[129] The National Institute of Neurological Disorders and Stroke rt-PA Stroke Study Group. (1995) Tissue plasminogen activator for acute ischemic stroke. *N Engl J Med* 333:1581-1587.

[130] Furlan A, Higashida R, Wechsler L, et al. (1999) Intra-arterial prourokinase for acute ischemic stroke. The PROACT II Study: a randomized controlled trial. *JAMA* 282:2003-2011.

[131] Tanne D, Kasner SE, Demchuk AM, et al. (2002) Markers of increased risk of intracerebral hemorrhage after intravenous recombinant tissue plasminogen activator therapy for acute ischemic stroke in clinical practice. *Circulation* 105:1679-1685.

[132] Mahaffey KW, Granger CB, Sloan MA, et al. (1998) Risk factors for in hospital nonhemorrhagic stroke in patients with acute myocardial infarction treated with thrombolysis: results from GUSTO-I. *Circulation* 97:757- 764.

[133] Warach S, Latour LL. (2004) Evidence of reperfusion injury, exacerbated by thrombolytic therapy, in human focal brain ischemia using a novel imaging marker of early blood-brain barrier disruption. *Stroke* 35:2659-2661.

[134] Mahaffey KW, Granger CB, Sloan MA, et al. (1999) Neurosurgical evacuation of intracranial hemorrhage after thrombolytic therapy for acute myocardial infarction: experience from the GUSTO-I trial. Global Utilization of Streptokinase and Tissue-plasminogen activator (tPA) for Occluded coronary arteries. *Am Heart J* 138:493- 499.

[135] Liu AC, Segaren N, Cox TS, et al. (2006) Is there a role for magnetic resonance imaging in the evaluation of non-traumatic intraparenchymal haemorrhage in children? *Pediatr Radiol* 36:940-946.

[136] Warren DL, JoEllen L, Jerome R, Elizabeth PE, Steve R. (2008) Intracranial Hemorrhage in Children An Evolving Spectrum. *Arch Neurol* 65:1629-1633.

[137] Jordan LC, Hillis AE. (2007) Hemorrhagic stroke in children. *Pediat Neurol* 36:73-80.

[138] Van Gijn J, Rinkel GJ. (2001) Subarachnoid haemorrhage: diagnosis, causes and management. *Brain* 124:249-278.

[139] Longstreth WT Jr, Nelson LM, Koepsell TD, van Belle G. (1993) Clinical course of spontaneous subarachnoid hemorrhage: a population-based study in King County, Washington. *Neurology* 43:712-718.

[140] Broderick JP, Brott TG, Duldner JE, Tomsick T, Leach A. (1994) Initial and recurrent bleeding are the major causes of death following subarachnoid hemorrhage. *Stroke* 25:1342-1347.

[141] Mayberg MR, Batjer HH, Dacey R, et al. (1994) Guidelines for the management of aneurysmal subarachnoid hemorrhage: a statement for healthcare professionals from a special writing group of the Stroke Council, American Heart Association. *Stroke* 25:2315-2328.

[142] Lindsay KW, Teasdale GM, Knill- Jones RP. (1983) Observer variability in assessing the clinical features of subarachnoid hemorrhage. *J Neurosurg* 58:57-62.

[143] Broderick JP, Brott T, Tomsick T, Huster G, Miller R. (1992) The risk of subarachnoid and intracerebral hemorrhages in blacks as compared with whites. *N Engl J Med* 326:733-736.

[144] Hijdra A, van Gijn J, Nagelkerke NJ, Vermeulen M, van Crevel H. (1988) Prediction of delayed cerebral ischemia, rebleeding, and outcome after aneurysmal subarachnoid hemorrhage. *Stroke* 19:1250-1256.

[145] Qureshi AI, Suri MF, Yahia AM, et al. (2001) Risk factors for subarachnoid hemorrhage. *Neurosurgery* 49:607-612.

[146] Broderick JP, Viscoli CM, Brott T, et al. (2003) Major risk factors for aneurysmal subarachnoid hemorrhage in the young are modifiable. *Stroke* 34:1375-1381.

[147] Teunissen LL, Rinkel GJ, Algra A, van Gijn J. (1996) Risk factors for subarachnoid hemorrhage: a systematic review. *Stroke* 27:544-549.

[148] Bambakidis NC, Selman WR. Subarachnoid hemorrhage. In: Suarez JI, ed. Critical care neurology and neurosurgery. Totowa, N.J.: Humana Press, 2004:365-377.

[149] Schievink WI, Michels VV, Piepgras DG. (1994) Neurovascular manifestations of heritable connective tissue disorders: a review. *Stroke* 25:889-903.

[150] Wiebers DO, Whisnant JP, Huston J III, et al. (2003) Unruptured intracranial aneurysms: natural history, clinical outcome, and risks of surgical a endovascular treatment. *Lancet*;362:103-110.

[151] White PM, Wardlaw J. (2003) Unruptured intracranial aneurysms: prospective data have arrived. *Lancet*;362:90-91.

[152] Hunt WE, Hess RM. (1968) Surgical risk as related to time of intervention in the repair of intracranial aneurysms. *J Neurosurg*;28:14-20.

[153] Report of World Federation of Neurological Surgeons committee on a universal subarachnoid hemorrhage grading scale. (1988) *J Neurosurg* 68:985-986.

[154] Fisher CM, Kistler JP, Davis JM. (1980) Relation of cerebral vasospasm to subarachnoid hemorrhage visualized by computed tomographic scanning. *Neurosurgery* 6:1-9.

[155] Claassen J, Bernardini GL, Kreiter K, et al. (2001) Effect of cisternal and ventricular blood on risk of delayed cerebral ischemia after subarachnoid hemorrhage: the Fisher scale revisited. *Stroke* 32:2012-2020.

[156] Edlow JA, Caplan LR. (2000) Avoiding pitfalls in the diagnosis of subarachnoid hemorrhage. *N Engl J Med* 342:29-36.

[157] Kowalski RG, Claassen J, Kreiter KT, et al. (2004) Initial misdiagnosis and outcome after subarachnoid hemorrhage. *JAMA* 291:866-869.

[158] Van der Jagt M, Hasan D, Bijvoet HW, et al. (1999) Validity of prediction of the site of ruptured intracranial aneurysms with CT. *Neurology* 52:34-39.

[159] Jayaraman MV, Mayo-Smith WW, Tung GA, et al. (2004) Detection of intracranial aneurysms: multi-detector row CT angiography compared with DSA. *Radiology*;230:510-518.

[160] Bardach NS, Olson SJ, Elkins JS, Smith WS, Lawton MT, Johnston SC. (2004) Regionalization of treatment for subarachnoid hemorrhage: a cost utility analysis. *Circulation* 109:2207-2212.

[161] Commichau C, Scarmeas N, Mayer SA. (2003) Risk factors for fever in the neurologic intensive care unit. *Neurology* 60:837-841.

[162] Dorhout Mees SM, van Dijk GW, Algra A, Kempink DR, Rinkel GJ. (2003) Glucose levels and outcome after subarachnoid hemorrhage. *Neurology* 61:1132-1133.

[163] Rinkel GJ, Feigin VL, Algra A, van den Bergh WM, Vermeulen M, Gijn J. (2005) Calcium antagonists for aneurysmal subarachnoid hemorrhage. *Cochrane Database Syst Rev* 1:CD000277.

[164] Roos YB, Rinkel GJ, Vermeulen M, Algra A, van Gijn J. (2003) Antifibrinolytic therapy for aneurysmal subarachnoid hemorrhage. *Cochrane Database Syst Rev* 2:CD001245.

[165] Whitfield PC, Kirkpatrick PJ. (2001)Timing of surgery for aneurismal subarachnoid hemorrhage. *Cochrane Database Syst Rev* 2:CD001697.

[166] Guglielmi G, Vinuela F, Dion J, Duckwiler G. (1991) Electrothrombosis of saccular aneurysms via endovascular approach. Part 2: preliminary clinical experience. *J Neurosurg* 75:8-14.

[167] Molyneux A, Kerr R, Stratton I, et al. (2002) International Subarachnoid Aneurysm Trial (ISAT) of neurosurgical clipping versus endovascular coiling in 2143 patients with ruptured intracranial aneurysms: a randomised trial. *Lancet* 360:1267-1274.

[168] Molyneux AJ, Kerr RS, Yu L-M, et al. (2005) International Subarachnoid Aneurysm Trial (ISAT) of neurosurgical clipping versus endovascular coiling in 2143 patients with ruptured intracranial aneurysms: a randomised comparison of effects on survival, dependency, seizures, rebleeding, subgroups, and aneurysm occlusion. *Lancet* 366:809-817.

[169] Johnston SC, Higashida RT, Barrow DL, Caplan LR, Dion JE, Hademenos G, Hopkins LN, Molyneux A, Rosenwasser RH, Vinuela F, Wilson CB. (2002) Recommendations for the endovascular treatment of intracranial aneurysms: a statement for healthcare professionals from the Committee on Cerebrovascular Imaging of the American Heart Association Council on Cardiovascular *Radiology* 33:2536-2544.

[170] Solenski NJ, Haley EC Jr, Kassell NF, et al. (1995) Medical complications of aneurysmal subarachnoid hemorrhage: a report of the multicenter, cooperative aneurysm study. *Crit Care Med* 23:1007-1017.

[171] Van Gijn J, Hijdra A, Wijdicks EF, Vermeulen M, van Crevel H. (1985) Acute hydrocephalus after aneurysmal subarachnoid hemorrhage. *J Neurosurg* 63:355-362.

[172] Alexandrov AV (Ed.). *Cerebrovascular ultrasound in stroke prevention and treatment.* New York: Blackwell Publishing 2004; 81-129.

[173] Fujiwara H, Oki K, Momoshima S. (2005) PROPELLER diffusion weighted magnetic resonance imaging of acute spinal epidural hematoma. *Acta Radiol* 46:539-542.

[174] Gouveia LO, Castanho P, Ferreira JJ, Guedes MM, Falcao F, e Melo TP. (2007) Chiropractic manipulation: reasons for concern?. *Clin Neurol Neurosurg* 109:922-925.

[175] Arrese I, Lobato RD, Gomez PA. (2004) Hyperacute epidural haematoma isodense with the brain on computed tomography. *Acta Neurochir (Wien)* 146:193-194.

[176] Bezircioglu H, Ersahin Y, Demircivi F, et al. (1996) Nonoperative treatment of acute extradural hematomas: analysis of 80 cases. *J Trauma* 41:696-698.

[177] De Souza M, Moncure M, Lansford T, Albaugh G, Tarnoff M, Goodman M, et al. (2007) Nonoperative management of epidural hematomas and subdural hematomas: is it safe in lesions measuring one centimeter or less?. *J Trauma* 63:370-372.

[178] Suzuki S, Endo M, Kurata A. (2004) Efficacy of endovascular surgery for the treatment of acute epidural hematomas. *AJNR Am J Neuroradiol* 25:1177-1180.

[179] Park J, Kim GJ, Hwang SK. (2008) Thrombolytic evacuation of post-craniotomy epidural haematomas using closed suction drains: a pilot study. *Acta Neurochi(Wien)* 150:359-366.

[180] Kotwica Z, Brzezinski J. (1993) Acute subdural haematoma in adults: an analysis of outcome in comatose patients. *Acta Neurochir (Wien)* 21:95-99.

[181] Suman S, Meenakshisundaram S, Woodhouse P. (2006) Bilateral chronic subdural haematoma: a reversible cause of parkinsonism. *J R Soc Med* 99:91-92.

[182] Bullock MR, Chesnut R, Ghajar J, Gordon D, Hartl R, Newell DW, et al. (2006) Surgical management of acute subdural hematomas. *Neurosurgery* 58:S16-24.

[183] Horn EM, Feiz-Erfan I, Bristol RE, Spetzler RF, Harrington TR. (2006) Bedside twist drill craniostomy for chronic subdural hematoma: a comparative study. *Surg Neurol* 65:150-153.

[184] Lollis SS, Wolak ML, Mamourian AC. (2006) Imaging characteristics of the subdural evacuating port system, a new bedside therapy for subacute/chronic subdural hematoma. *AJNR Am J Neuroradiol* 27:74-75.

[185] Aminoff MJ. (1987) Vascular disorders of the spinal cord. In: Davidoff RA, ed. *Handbook of the Spinal Cord*. New York: Marcel Dekker :259-297.

[186] Geldmacher DS, Bowen BC. Spinal cord vascular disease. (2004) In: Bradley WG, Daroff RB, Fenichel GM, Marsden CD, eds. *Neurology in Clinical Practice Principles of Diagnosis and Management.* 4th ed. Philadelphia, Pa: Butterworth-Heimann:1313-1322.

Groen RJM. (2004) Non-operative treatment of spontaneous spinal epidural hematomas: a review of the literature and a comparison with operative cases. *Acta Neurochir (Wien)* 146:103-110.

In: Hematomas: Types, Treatments … ISBN: 978-1-61942-385-5
Editors: M.F.G.Salazar…pp. 79-120

Chapter III

Infected Hematomas: Review of the Literature

Pilar López García
Microbiology Laboratory
Public Hospital Elche HGU (Alicante), Spain

1. Abstract

The infected hematomas are clinical slightly frequent entities or that in rare occasions have been communicated in the literature and therefore with an unknown morbidity-mortality. Probably some infected hematomas have been communicated in the shape of abscesses in different locations. The clinical expression of the entity is diverse and his diagnosis can turn out to be difficult. The diagnostic image technologies and the samples for the microbiological studies allow the diagnosis and precocious beginning of the treatment and the reduction of the morbidity-mortality. On having done a review of the bibliography (bibliometric search realized essentially in the MEDLINE database, using PubMed search interface), they find isolated cases and few series with scanty patients with infected hematomas. The bacteria isolated with major frequency have been *Escherichia coli*, different kinds of anaerobic, *Staphylococcus aureus*, *Salmonella sp*, *Mycoplasma hominis* and *Streptococcus pneumoniae*. The infected cranial hematomas have been more frequently described followed by those of abdominal location.

2. Introduction

The infected hematomas are clinical slightly frequent entities or that in scanty occasions have been communicated in the literature and therefore with an unknown morbidity-mortality. Probably some infected hematomas have been communicated in the shape of abscesses or empyemas in different locations. The clinical expression of this entity changes according to the subjects, the affected organs and the responsible microorganisms. His diagnosis can turn out to be difficult for his scanty symptomatology, insidious appearance or for being confused with tumors or other pathologies. In the bibliography there meet isolated cases and series of few patients with infected hematomas.

3. Material and Methods

A bibliometric search has been realized until August, 2011 in the database MEDLINE, using PubMed search interface [1,2,3,4,5,6,7,8,9,10...]. They looked terms were: hematoma, hematoma and infection, infected hematoma, spontaneous infected hematoma, hematoma and empyema, infection and empyema, hematoma and abscess, muscular hematoma and infection, spontaneous muscular hematoma and infection, subdural hematoma, subdural hematoma and empyema, subdural infection, epidural hematoma and infection, subgaleal hematoma and infection, liver hematoma and infection, subcapsular hepatic hematoma and infection, etc. The epidemiological, clinical characteristics and the microbiological etiology of the infected hematomas communicated in the literature are checked. Also there has been checked, by means of other seekers, the bibliography related to some of the previous terms.

4. Hematoma: Definition. Infected Hematoma

A hematoma is an accumulation of blood confined in a space, caused by the break of capillary glasses, which appears generally as corporal resultant response at one stroke or in occasions of spontaneous form. If the patient takes anticoagulants it is probably that he presents hematomas easier. The hematoma can become infected. The route of infection can be hematogenous seeding, or for direct irruption of the microorganisms: contiguous infection, perforation of infected or colonized organs, traumatism, etc.

5. Types of Hematomas

The hematomas often are described on the basis of his location. They can develop in the skin and also in the internal organs, being the most dangerous those that happen inside the cranium. This way so according to the affected zone they qualify in: *subcutaneous* hematomas, located under the skin; *Intramuscular*: inside the protuberant part of the underlying muscle. The muscular hematomas are in the habit of being masses limited generally to the only muscle. The intramuscular hematomas [6,10,27,75,91] can be very painful. Some muscles are surrounded by bands of hard fabrics and if the bled one is important, the pressure inside these compartments can increase and produce a "compartment syndrome". In this situation, the supply of blood of the muscle meets awkward and the muscles and other structures like the nerves can be damaged of permanent form. This is observed more commonly in the leg and the forearm. Nevertheless the inter or intramuscular (10) infected hematomas are very scanty described. In the checked literature they are described *epidural*, *subdural* [2,5,4,8,12,13,21,22,23,24,25,26,29, 36,37,40,44,54,55,59,60,65,67,68,70,72,74,76,77,86,95,100,103,105,110,111, 116,119], *subarachnoid, subgaleal* [20,39], and *cerebral* [16,30,49,52,120](due to the bled one of the arterial pressure discharge, an escape or break of aneurysm, trauma, tumor or a cerebral hemorrhage) infected hematomas. The *cephalohematomas* are frequent in children [4,9,17,42, 46,47,58,63,66,80,93,109,112,113,115,]. Likewise *scalp* [50, 102,], *ear, face,* [114] *orbital* [117], *retropharyngeal* [19] and *nasal* hematomas become infected. The orthopedic injuries associate often with formation of hematomas. The *bones* associate almost always with hematomas in the site of fracture. The fractures of the long bones like femur and the top part of the humerus can be associated with the bled one importantly. The fractures of the bony pelvis also can cause a considerable hematoma since it is difficult to control the hemorrhage in this zone. The pelvic hematomas can be difficult to diagnose. *Periosteum* and *pericondra*l hematomas have been described. The *subungueal* hematomas are the result of the injuries of the top of the fingers. In the skin there take place equimosis due to a traumatism or injuries in the blood superficial glasses in the skin. The persons who take anticoagulative treatment are more susceptible to subcutaneous hematomas. Infected *wounds* *hematomas* [3,84], scanty *thoracic* [18,69], *mediastinal* [71,106], *intrapulmonary* [18,97] infected hematomas associate to maneuvers of resuscitation; abscess and diverse traumatism have been communicated. In the *intraabdominal* [82,106] location the hemorrhage can owe to a variety of injuries or diseases: bruise peritoneal (ex. in peritonitis), *retroperitoneal* hematoma [62,104] and in other abdominal locations: abdominal muscles, abdominal wall [27,45,57,83,85,94], epigastria [43], etc (82]. The hematoma also can take place in *adrenal* [51,90] location, solid organs as *spleen* [11,33,88], *kidney* [28,53,64,99], *liver* [15,31,34,41,61,73,78,81,87], or in the bed of these last two organs in case of transplant [28]. They can take place inside the walls of the small and or thick *intestine.* During the menstruation they can produce clots that are accumulated in the *vagina.* Also clots of blood can be formed after the childbirth. It is not normal bled vaginal during the pregnancy and must be a motive of medical consultation. *Pelvic* [14,107], *Ovaric* [108], *chorionic* [89], *subchorionic* infected hematomas and in cases of sutures for Caesarean and after *genitourinary tract surgery* [48,56,96,118.] *Extravascular* infected hematomas [79,98,101] and others are listed. *Table 1.(PUBMED), Table 2* and *Graphic 1.*

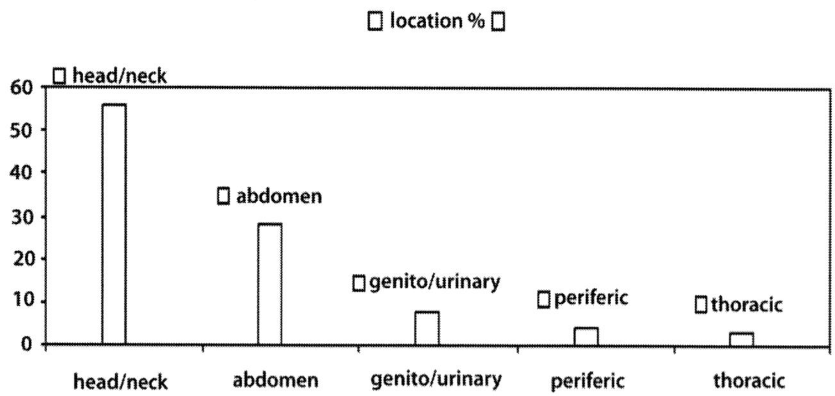

Graphic 1. Hematomas location.

Table 1. Infected hematomas: Review of the literature

Article	Publication Year/Author	Cases	Sex Age group	Age	Pathology	Microorganism
Head and neck hematomas						
Cerebral fungal infection with mycotic aneurysm of basilar artery and subarachnoid hemorrhage	2009 Ahsan H	A case	man	28 y	aneurysm	*Aspergillus sp.*
Four cases of the infectious cerebral aneurysms	2004 Oshita J	4 cases	1 man 2 woman's 1 woman	60 y 71+71 y 49 y	Endocarditis	
Neuritis of the nervus infraorbitalis caused by an infected hematoma after tuberal anesthesia	1954 Dhom H	A case			Tuberal anesthesia	
Retropharyngeal infected hematoma: a unique complication of nasogastric tube insertion	2009 Hirshoren N	A case			nasogastric tube insertion	
Intracerebral hematoma complicated with brain abscess in an infant. Case report	2008 Eser O	A case	1 infant	45 d	Intracerebral hematoma x vitamin K deficiency	
Unusual Infected hematoma: report of case	1969 Ewbank RL	A case			Dental pathology	

Table 1. (Continued).

Article	Publication Year/Author	Cases	Sex Age group	Age	Pathology	Microorganism
Head and neck : *Subdural and epidural hematomas*						
Pyogenic abscess from *Providencia stuartii* mimicking necrotic tumor at perfusion-weighted imaging	2011 Muccio CF	A case	woman	74 y	Postsurgical subdural hematoma	*Providencia stuartii*
Infected acute subdural hematoma associated with invasive pneumococcal disease.	2011 Kagami H	A case	woman	68 y	Cranial traumatism+ Pneumonia +Meningitis	*Streptococcus pneumoniae*
Chronic subdural empyema and cranial vault osteomyelitis due to *Salmonella paratyphi A*	2010 Bhooshan P	A case	man	42 y	Cranial traumatism	*Salmonella paratyphi* A
Empyema of preexisting subdural hemorrhage caused by a rare Salmonella species after in a foster home	2010 Tabarani CM	A case	infant		exposure to bearded dragons	*Salmonella enterica* subspecies houtenae (IV) serotype 44:z4,z23
Infantile chronic subdural hematoma infected by *Escherichia coli*-case report	2010 Iimura Y	A case	child	6 m	Without pathological precedents	*Escherichia coli*

Article	**Publication Year/Author**	**Cases**	**Sex Age group**	**Age**	**Pathology**	**Microorganism**
Infected subdural haematoma due to *Salmonella enterica* serovar *Typhimurium* in an adult	**2010 Hayakawa K**	A case	man	65 y	Alcoholism + gastrectomia	*Salmonella typhimurium*
Chronic subdural hematoma infected by *Salmonella*	2009 Aslan A	A case	girl	6 m		*Salmonella typhi*
Case of infected subdural hematoma diagnosed by diffusion-weighted imaging	2009 Narita E	A case	man	80 y	Gastrectomía+ Cranial traumatism	*Escherichia coli*
Salmonella-Infected Chronic Subdural Hematoma	2009 Adem A	A case	man	55 y	Alcoholism +Chronic Subdural hematoma	*Salmonella thypi*
Infected subdural hematoma in an infant	2008 Hoshina T	A case	child	1 y	Subdural hematoma	*Streptococcus pneumoniae*
Spinal subdural haematoma: a rare complication of low-molecular-weight heparin therapy.	2008 Chau SY	A case	man	52 y	heparin therapy	*Salmonella parathyphi*
Fatal cerebritis and brain abscesses following a nontraumatic subdural hematoma in a chronic hemodialyzed patient	2008 Mesquita M	A case	man	65 y	Hemodialysis +Bacteriemia	*Staphylococcus aureus*

Table 1. (Continued).

Article	Publication Year/Author	Cases	Sex Age group	Age	Pathology	Microorganism
Case of bilateral subdural empyema complicating *Campylobacter fetus subspecies fetus* meningitis	2008 Kanayama S	A case	man	51 y	Meningitis	*Campylobacter fetus subspecies fetus*
Pneumocephalus from gas-forming *Escherichia coli* subdural empyema	2007 Adamides AA	A case				*Escherichia coli*
Subdural empyema caused by an unusual organism following intracranial haematoma	2007 Le Roux PC	A case	man	6 y	gastroenteritis	*Salmonella spp*
A case of infected subdural hematoma	2007 Otsuka T	A case	man	87 y	Chronic subdural hematoma	
Infected and calcified chronic subdural hematoma presenting an attitude of acute hematoma on MRI: case report	2005 Sato K	A case	Man	50 y	Without pathological precedents	
Mycoplasma hominis infection of a subdural haematoma in the peripartum period	2003 Douglas MW	A case			childbirth	*Mycoplasma hominis*

Article	Publication Year/Author	Cases	Sex Age group	Age	Pathology	Microorganism
Infectious endocarditis associated with subarachnoid haemorrhage, subdural hematoma and multiple brain abscesses	2003 Yanagihara C	A case	man	54 y	Infectious Endocarditis+ intracerebral hemorrhage + +subdural hematoma +cerebral abscess	*Staphylococcus aureus*
Ruptured infectious aneurysm of the distal middle cerebral artery manifesting as intracerebral hemorrhage and acute subdural hematoma-case report	2003 Yamakawa H	A case	woman	21 y	Infectious endocarditis	
A case of infected subdural hematoma following chronic subdural hematoma irrigation	2002 Honda M	A case	woman	71 y	Parkinson Diabetes Mellitus Urinary Infection	*Klebsiella pneumoniae*
A case of infected subdural hematoma due to *Campylobacter fetus*	2001 Ishii N	A case	woman	20 y	slightly cooked liver+ cranial traumatism	*Campylobacter fetus*
Subdural empyema due to *Mycoplasma hominis* following epidural anesthesia	2000 Escamilla F	A case	woman	32 y	Caesarean.	*Mycoplasma hominis*

Table 1. (Continued).

Article	Publication Year/Author	Cases	Sex Age group	Age	Pathology	Microorganism
A case of infected subdural hematoma	1998 Sawauchi S	A case	woman	77 y	Chronic subdural Hematoma + urinary infection	*Escherichia coli*
Subdural empyema caused by hematogenous dissemination from an abscess in thigh to a preexisting chronic subdural hematoma—case report	1998 Kawamoto S	A case	man	63 y	SARM bacteriemia from thigh	*Staphylococcus aureus* (SARM)
A case of infected subdural hematoma complicating chronic subdural hematoma in a healthy adult man	1997 Yamasaki F	A case	man	55 y	Traffic accident+ chronic subdural hematoma +bacteriemia	*Enterococcus faecalis*
Infected subdural effusion associated with resolving subdural hematoma--case report	1997 Aoki N	A case	man	70 y	Traumatism+subdural hematoma	*Campylobacter fetus*
Primary *Candida albicans* empyema associated with epidural hematomas in craniocervical junction	1997 Duffner F	A case	man	27 y	Craniocervical empyema	*Candida albicans*

Article	**Publication Year/Author**	**Cases**	**Sex Age group**	**Age**	**Pathology**	**Microorganism**
Subdural abscess following chronic subdural hematoma	1995 Hirano A	A case	man	86 y	Chronic subdural hematoma + cholecystitis +bacteriemia	*Escherichia coli*
Spinal subdural abscess. Case report	1992 Bartels RH	A case				*Escherichia coli*
Subdural empyema caused by *Escherichia coli*: hematogenous dissemination to a preexisting chronic subdural hematoma	1995 Bakker S	A case			Chronic subdural hematoma+ bacteriemia	*Escherichia coli*
Infected chronic subdural hematoma due to an ethmoiditis; a case report	1989 Itoh S	A case			Chronic subdural hematoma + ethmoiditis	
Encapsulated subdural empyema--a case report with special reference to CT findings and operative indications	1985 Tokunaga Y	A case	child	18 m	Cranial traumatism	
Pasteurella multocida subdural empyema: a case report	1981 Khan MI	A case			bacteriemia	*Pasteurella multocida*

Table 1. (Continued).

Article	Publication Year/Author	Cases	Sex Age group	Age	Pathology	Microorganism
Infected subdural hematoma: three case reports involving gram-negative organisms	1975 Vertrovec GW	3 cases			Bacteriemia + Infected Subdural hematoma	*Escherichia coli* (1case) *Salmonella spp* (2cases)
Salmonella-infected subdural hematoma	1972 Lerner PI	A case				*Salmonella spp*
Infected subdural hematoma	1967 Geetter DM	A case				
Subdural empyema probably secondary to infected chronic subdural hematoma; case report	1949 Klos HJ	A case				
Head and neck : *Cephalohematomas, Subgaleal hematomas, Scalp and skull hematomas*						
Septicemia, meningitis, and skull osteomyelitis complicating infected cephalhematoma caused by ESBL-producing *Escherichia coli*	2011 Nakwan N	A case	newborn		cephalohematoma	*E coli* BLEE

Article	Publication Year/Author	Cases	Sex Age group	Age	Pathology	Microorganism
Escherichia coli meningitis and parietal osteomyelitis in an infant: a rare complication of cephalohematoma	2010 Van Helleputte C	A case	Child	30 d	Fetal monitoring	*Escherichia coli*
Escherichia coli- infected cephalohematoma in an infant	2009 Weiss KJ	A case	girl	1 m	Cephalohematoma + Bacteriemia + meningitis	*Escherichia coli*
MRI features of an infected cephalohaematoma in a neonate	2006 Chen MH	A case	neonate	23 d	Cephalohematoma + bacteriemia	*Escherichia coli*
Infected neonatal cephalohematomas caused by anaerobic bacteria	2005 Brook L	6 cases	neonates		Vacuum, Amnionitis, fetal monitoring, long childbirth (2-4 microorganism /patient) Anaerobic +- aerobic bacteria	*Peptostreptococcus* 5, *Prevotella* 4 *B.fragilis* 2, *Propionibacterium acnes* 1, *Escherichia coli, Staphylococcus aureus, Steptoc.beta h. B*

Table 1. (Continued).

Article	Publication Year/Author	Cases	Sex Age group	Age	Pathology	Microorganism
Infected cephalohematoma of newborns: experience in a medical center in Taiwan	2005 Chang HY	28 cases	newborns		cephalohematomas	57% *Ecoli* (n16) 18% *Staphylococcus aureus* (n5) 36% others
Infected cephalohematoma associated with sepsis and scalp cellulitis: a case report	2002 Fan HC	A case	newborn		cephalohematoma	*Escherichia coli*
Spontaneously infected cephalohematoma: case report and review of the literature. Discussion	2000 Goodwin MD	A case			cephalohematoma	
Infected cephalohematoma associated with sepsis and skull osteomyelitis: report of one case	1999 Kao HC	A case	boy	37 d	sepsis	*Escherichia coli*
Infected cephalohematoma associated with Osteomyelitis, sepsis and meningitis	1993 Blom NA	A case	child		Cephalo-hematoma	
Cephalohematoma infection in neonatal septicemia	1989 Meignier M	A case	neonate		Septicemia+ meningitis	

Article	**Publication Year/Author**	**Cases**	**Sex Age group**	**Age**	**Pathology**	**Microorganism**
Isolation of *Salmonella typhimurium* from cephalohematoma and osteomyelitis	1978 Diwan N	A case			Cephalo-hematoma	*Salmonella typhimurium*
Infected cephalohaematoma	1972 Chan MC	A case			Cephalo-hematoma	
Cephalohematoma infected with *Bacteroides*	1971 Lee Y	A case			Cephalo-hematoma	*Bacteroides spp*
Bacteremia, infected cephalohematoma, and osteomyelitis of the skull in a newborn	1967 Levy HL	A case	newborn		Cephalo-hematoma	
Late onset subgaleal haemorrhage infection with *Streptococcus pneumoniae*	2009 Slap F	A case	child	11 m	Otitis	*Streptococcus pneumoniae*
Cephalic injury of soft parts in one Child of months	2008 Jimeno A	A case	child	9 m	subgaleal abscess	*Streptococcus pneumoniae*
Infected subgaleal hematoma in a neonate	2007 Pollack S	A case	neonate		subgaleal hematoma	Polymicrobial (+ anaerobic bacteria)
Gardnerella vaginalis-infected scalp hematoma associated with electronic fetal monitoring	2004 Eggink BH	A case	neonate		fetal monitoring	*Gardnerella vaginalis*

Table 1. (Continued).

Article	Publication Year/Author	Cases	Sex Age group	Age	Pathology	Microorganism
Infected scalp hematoma	1983 Handrick W	A case	neonate		Cephalo-hematoma post vacuum	*Escherichia coli*
Thoracic hematomas						
Chronic expanding hematoma with bronchopleural fistula and empyema space	2009 Tsubochi H	A case	Man	65 y	bronchopleural fistula + TBC	*Enterococcus casseliflavus*
A case of intrathoracic chronic expanding hematoma	1998 Mori S	A case	woman	69 y	TBC + pneumotorax	¿*Mycobacterium tuberculosis*?
Mediastinal abscesses and empyema of the pleural cavity after iatrogenic fracture of the sternum	1997 Kaminski Z	A case	Man	68 a	Iatrogenic fracture	
Radiologic case of the month. Pneumatocele on infected intrapulmonary hematoma	1988 Alembik Y	A case			Pulmonary hematoma	
Abdominal cavity, abdominal organs and muscles hematomas						

Article	**Publication Year/Author**	**Cases**	**Sex Age group**	**Age**	**Pathology**	**Microorganism**
Postoperative infection of an epigastria hematoma caused by *Aeromonas veronii* biovar *sobria*	2006 Bomke AK	A case	Man	52 y	Postoperative gastric carcinoma	*Aeromonas veronii* biovar *sobria sobria*
Iliopsoas hematoma consequent to prosthetic graft infection with methicillin resistant *Staphylococcus aureus* in a hemodialysis patient	2008 Abe M	A case			Hemodialysis+ prostethic graft	*Staphylococcus aureus* SARM
Infected rectus hematoma simulating an appendiceal abscess on CT scan	2007 Tranchart H	A case				
Psoas abscess: report of a series and review of the literature	2005 Van den Berge M	12 cases (a case infected Hemat.)			Hemopylia + psoas abscesses+ infected hematoma	*Staphylococcus aureus*
Hematomas of the abdominal rectus muscle	1993 Fusato G	12 cases (1 case infected hemat.)				
Infected intraabdominal hematomes: percutaneous drainage	1993 García-Vila J	5 cases				

Table 1. (Continued).

Article	Publication Year/Author	Cases	Sex Age group	Age	Pathology	Microorganism
Abdominal wall hematoma	1992 Andersen E	A case			Tuberculosis	*Mycobacterium tuberculosis*
Rectus abdominis sheath hematoma as a complication of tetanus. Diagnosis by computed tomography scanning	1989 Suhr GM	A case			Tetanus	*Clostridium tetanii*
Abdominal cavity, abdominal organs and muscles hematomas: ***Liver hematomas***						
A case of liver abscess with subcapsular hematoma mimicking ruptured hepatic cholangiocarcinoma	2009 Kim CH	A case	Man	59 y	Liver abscess	
Hepatic subcapsular hematoma after CPRE	2007 Priego P	A case	man	35 y	Coledoco-lithiasis	*Escherichia coli*
Abdominal pain and fever after CPRE: hepatic hematoma after CPRE	2007 Mongil LL	A case			CPRE	*Escherichia coli + Bacteroides spp*

Article	Publication Year/Author	Cases	Sex Age group	Age	Pathology	Microorganism
Infected hepatic hematoma after renal extracorporeal shock wave lithotripsy	2006 Neto AC	A case	woman	35 y	lithotriosy	*Klebsiella spp*
Subcapsular liver hematoma	2001 Triki A	2 cases (1 infected h.)				
Intrahepatic hematoma with secondary *Salmonella* infection via biliary fistula.	1997 Cerwenka H	A case			biliar reservoir + hepatic traumatism	*Salmonella spp.*
Liver abscess following blunt trauma: a case report and review of the literature	1994 Haight DO	A case	man	32 y	Traumatism	*Haemophilus paraphrophilus*
Mycoplasma hominis in liver transplantation	1993 Haller M	A case			Liver transplantation	*Mycoplasma hominis*
Mycoplasma hominis infection of perihepatic hematomas in a liver transplant recipient	1992 Jacobs F	A case			Transplant recipient	*Mycoplasma hominis*
Abdominal cavity, abdominal organs and muscles hematomas ***Renal, peri-renal and Retroperitoneal hemat.***						

Table 1. (Continued).

Article	**Publication Year/Author**	**Cases**	**Sex Age group**	**Age**	**Pathology**	**Microorganism**
Transcatheter embolization of an isolated lumbar arterial bleeding complicating radical nephrectomy for renal infarction with infected peri-renal hematoma a	2008 Geldof K	A case				
Clostridium innocuum bacteremia secondary to infected hematoma with gas formation in a kidney transplant recipient	2003 Castiglioni B	A case	woman	38 y	VHC + transplant recipient	*Clostridium innocuum*
¿ How should an infected perinephric haematoma be drained in a tetraplegic patient with baclofen pump implanted in the abdominal wall?	2002 Vaidyanatha n S	A case	man	56 y	tetraplegic patient + warfarine	multiresistent *Pseudomonas aeruginosa*
Hematoma infection with *Mycoplasma hominis* following transplant nephrectomy	2000 Legg JM	A case	man	18 y	transplant nephrectomy	*Mycoplasma hominis*

Article	**Publication Year/Author**	**Cases**	**Sex Age group**	**Age**	**Pathology**	**Microorganism**
Wound and perinephric haematoma infection with *Mycoplasma hominis* in a renal transplant recipient	1993 Orange GV	A case			Transplant recipient	*Mycoplasma hominis*
Transcatheter intracavitary fibrinolysis of infected extravascular hematomas	1987 Vogelzang RL	2 cases	2 man	66 y 67 y	Prostate carcinoma surgery Renal carcinoma surgery	
Infected renal hematoma complicating anticoagulant therapy	1987 Morduchowicz G	A case			Warfarina therapy	
Infected retroperitoneal traumatic hematoma	1983 Loup J	A case			traumatism	
Superinfection of posttraumatic retroperitoneal hematoma secondary to ascending urinary tract infection	2001 Montravers P	A case			Renal traumatism + Urinary infection	
Infection of a traumatic pelvic hematoma with *Mycoplasma hominis*	1978 Burke DS	A case	Young man		Renal hematoma+ Pelvic traumatism	*Mycoplasma hominis*

Table 1. (Continued).

Article	Publication Year/Author	Cases	Sex Age group	Age	Pathology	Microorganism
Abdominal cavity, abdominal organs and muscles hematomas: ***Splenic hematomas***						
Splenic hematoma as a first manifestation of *Cytomegalovirus*	2010 Brncić N	A case	woman	44 y	Mononucleosis Syndrome	*Cytomegalovirus*
A rare case of infected splenic hematoma	2007 Godkar D	A case	man		Intravenous drug abuse+ endocarditis	
Salmonella C1 abscess in a Splenic hematoma	1992 Redondo Granado MJ	A case	child			*Salmonella C1*
Adrenal hematomas						
Bilateral neonatal adrenal abscess. Report of two cases and review of the literature	2003 Arena F	2 cases	Neon.		Adrenal abscess+ bacteriemia	
Adrenal abscess in the newborn: a case report and review of the literature	1990 Lizardo-Barahona JR	A case	New-born		calcified right adrenal hemorrhage	*Proteus mirabilis*

Article	Publication Year/Author	Cases	Sex Age group	Age	Pathology	Microorganism
Non-surgical drainage of intra-abdominal and mediastinal abscesses: a report of twelve cases	1981 Karlson KB	12 cases (1 adrenal infected hemat.)				
Genital, urinary, pelvic and gluteal hematomas						
Hematoma and abscess formation caused by *Mycoplasma hominis* following cesarean section	2011 Koshiba H	A case	woman	27 y	hematoma and abscess after cesarean section	*Mycoplasma hominis*
Severe pneumonia-peritoneum caused by infected pelvic hematoma: report of a case and review of the literature.	2010 Cui H	A case	Man	43 y	Postsurgical/ Cancer	*Bacteroides fragilis*
Obturator infected hematoma and urethral erosion following transobturator tape implantation. Transobturador	2004 Game X	A case				
Infected hematoma following tension-free vaginal tape implantation	2002 Neuman M	A case				
Gluteal hematoma infected with multiresistant *Salmonella typhi*	1997 Lindberg JA	A case				*Salmonella typhi*

Table 1. (Continued).

Article	Publication Year/Author	Cases	Sex Age group	Age	Pathology	Microorganism
Infected chorionic hematoma as a cause of infection in the 2nd trimester	1992 Weigel M	3 cases	3 pregnant woman's		Subchorionic hematoma	
Hematoma infected with *Mycoplasma hominis*	1988 Kailath EJ	A case	Young woman		Pelvic traumatism	*Mycoplasma hominis*
An infected ovarian hematoma as the presenting symptom of systemic lupus erythematosus	1978 Gleichner N	A case	woman		systemic lupus erythematosus + coagulation defect	
Two cases of infected hematoma of the broad ligament after low transverse caesarean section	1953 Guilhem P	2 cases	2 women´s		Caesarean section	
Peripheral arteries and muscles hematomas						
Infection of a spontaneous muscular hematoma due to *Robinsoniella peoriensis*, in a patient with alcoholic liver cirrhosis	2010 López P	A case	man	50 y	Alcoholic liver cirrhosis+ Coagulation defect+ femoral arterial rupture + muscle hematoma	*Robinsoniella peoriensis*

Article	**Publication Year/Author**	**Cases**	**Sex Age group**	**Age**	**Pathology**	**Microorganism**
Spontaneous bacterial seeding of a biceps hematoma	2010 Daney B.	A case	man	19 y	traumatism	*Streptococcus intermedius*
Blunt force injuries due to martial arts in children--a diagnostic problem? Delayed diagnosis of an infected hematoma	2010 Kruppa C	A case	child	9 y	Blunt force injuries	*Staphylococcus aureus*
Infected false aneurysm after puncture of an aneurysm of the deep femoral artery	1994 Berry MC	A case			postcatheter	*Staphylococcus aureus*
Infected false aneurysm of the deep femoral artery	1985 Gubko AA	A case				

Table 2. Hematomas: Locations

Head Neck 57%	Abdomen 28%	genital/ urinary 8%	Periphery 4 %	thoracic 3%
Cerebral	cavity	vagina	periphery artery	Mediast.
Subdural	muscles	chorionic	periphery muscles	lung
Cephaloh.	liver	subchorionic	others	
Subgaleal	kidney	caesarean		
Scalp	splendid	ovary		
others	adrenal			
	Retro-peritoneal	urinary tract		

6. Pathogeny. Underlying Pathologies and Routes of Infection

The injury of the vascular system causes the exit of the blood out of the vascular system. Since response to this situation starts a set of biological processes that try to control the hemorrhage (homeostasis). The homeostasis tends to obtain the formation of a resistant clot that closes the solution of continuity and stops the exit of the blood and depends on the interactions between vascular wall, nervous local reflections and substances liberated by the traumatic action, between them the serotonin, the platelets, which were forming the thrombus, and the concentration of a great quantity of plasmatic factors. To this a complex system is added of physiological inhibition and mechanisms of control that allow delimiting any excessive or inadequate activation of the haemostatic process.

The hemorrhages can be due to faults in the mechanism of the natural or spontaneous homeostasis, hereditary faults and acquired faults (infectious diseases purple and other purples), vascular alteration, platelet faults, surgical procedures, and or treatments with aspirin or other medicines with anticoagulative effect.

In the immunocompetent patient the response of the macrophages takes place to the presence of the microorganisms, beginning the recruitment of leukocytes and monocits to eliminate the microorganisms. This inflammatory response might stimulate the processes of the coagulation and the formation of fibrin to delimit the area of infection. The human body is specially sensitive to the bacterial endotoxines. In case of sepsis linked it produces a severe homeostasis alteration [33,38].

This way so the underlying pathology of the infected hematomas is of diverse nature: anticoagulant medicines [99], blood alterations, iatrogenic [19,31,34,41,117] (surgery, anesthetic technologies, and or diagnostic technologies), traumatisms [7,104], intra and extracranial pathologies , abdominal, thoracic pathologies, childbirth problems or caesarean [3,118], after septic processes (primary or secondary bacteriemia, sepsis ...) [2,93], contiguous infections (meningitis, abscesses, otitis, sinusitis, ethmoiditis ...) [25,39,77,95], cellulitis, endocarditis, osteomielitis, gastrointestinal infections, colecistitis, infections of the urinary tract [62], etc.

Frequently related to infected hematomas have been the anticoagulants, alcoholism, gastrectomia (both entities related often to infections by *Salmonella sp*) [13,103], bacteriemia, sepsis, meningitis, previous surgery, etc. The infections of intracranial hematomas, especially the subdurals and especially in small children, generally constitute complications of meningitis and other times are infections acquired by hematógen spread [8,17,26,100.]In major children and adult they are in the habit of being complications of sinusitis and infections of average ear, [20,39,95]. In all the groups of age they associate with procedures as craniotomies and chirugics procedures [21]. The related microorganisms more frequently with subdural infected hematoma are: *Escherichia coli* [8] and *Salmonella sp* [22]. Being the original area of infection the urinary and gastrointestinal tract.

7. Microbiological Etiology

The microorganism isolated with major frequency have been *Escherichia coli*, different kinds of anaerobic, *Salmonella sp*, *Staphylococcus aureus, Mycoplasma hominis* and *Streptococcus pneumoniae*. It is called the attention the frequent association of bruise infected by *Mycoplasma hominis* (54,64,65,81,84,87,96,107] spread by hematogenouse spread. Must be discard this microorganism specially in cases of infections which point of item could be an genital or urinary infection. This microorganism must be considered especially in transplanted patients, in immunologic pathology, in pelvic traumatism and gynecological, obstetric and urology's procedures, especially in hematomas with ordinary negative cultures.

Other microorganism identified are: *Streptococcus B beta hemolytic*, *Streptococcus intermedius*, *Enterococcus faecalis*, *Enterococcus casseliflavus*,

Klebsiella pneumoniae y *Klebsiella sp.*, *Proteus mirabilis*, *Providencia stuartii*, *Aeromonas veronii sobria*, *Pasteurella multocida*, *Campylobacter fetus fetus*, *Pseudomonas aeruginosa*, *Gardnerella vaginalis*, *Haemophilus paraprophilus*, *Mycobacterium tuberculosis*, *Aspergillus sp*, *Candida albicans and Cytomegalovirus.* In newborn cephalohematomas the predominant microorganisms have been *Escherichia coli*, *Staphylococcus aureus* and in the spinal hematomas *Staphylococcus aureus, b*eing also this microorganism the more frequent cause of bacteriemia and infected hematoma in hemodyalisis patients. Tables 3 and 4.

Table 3.

Identified microorganisms (%)	
Escherichia coli	28%
Anaerobic.	17%
Salmonella spp	11%
Staphylococcus aureus	10%
Mycoplasma hominis	9%
Streptococcus pneumoniae	4%
Campylobacter fetus fetus	<3%
Streptococcus spp	<2%
Enterococcus sp.	<2%
Klebsiella sp.	<2%
Mycobacterium tuberculosis	<2%
Aeromonas sobria	<1%
Pasteurella multocida	<1%
Proteus mirabilis	<1%
Providencia stuartii	<1%
Gardnerella vaginalis	<1%
Pseudomonas aeruginosa	<1%
Haemophilus paraphropilus	<1%
Aspergillus sp	<1%
Candida albicans	<1%
Cytomegalovirus	<1%

Table 4. Identified microorganisms (n)

Microorganisms			**total**
Staphylococcus aureus 10	*St. aureus* Methicilin resistant (SARM) 2		12
Streptococcus	*Streptococcus intermedius* 1	*Streptococcus beta h. B* 1	2
Streptococcus pneumoniae 5			5
Enterococcus	*Enterococcus faecalis* 1	*Enterococcus casseliflavus* 1	2
Escherichia coli 31	*E coli* Blee 1		32
Klebsiella	*Klebsiella pneumoniae* 1	*Klebsiella sp* 1	2
Proteus mirabilis 1			1
Providencia stuartii 1			1
Salmonella	*Salmonella spp* 6	Other spp. *Salmonella typhimurium* 2 *Salmonella San diego* 1 *Salmonella parathypi* 2 *Salmonella C1* 1 *Salmonella typhi* 2	14
Aeromonas veronii sobria 1			1
Campylobacter fetus fetus 3			3
Pasteurella multocida 1			1
Pseudomonas aeruginosa 1 multiresistent			1
Gardnerella vaginalis 1			1
Mycoplasma hominis 10			10
Anaerobic	Anaerobic others 2	*Robinsoniella peoriensis* 1 *Peptostreptococcus sp.* 5 *Prevotella sp.* 4 *Bacteroides fragilis* 3 *Bacteroides spp* 2 *Propionibacterium acnes* 1 *Clostridium tetanii* 1 *Clostridium innocuum* 1	20
Mycobacterium tuberculosis 2			2
Haemophilus paraprophilus 1			1
Cytomegalovirus 1			1
Aspergillus spp 1			1
Candida albicans 1			1

8. Diagnostics. Microbiological Diagnostics

The presumptive diagnosis by means of a clinical exhaustive history, being important the anamnesis of the familiar, personal precedents, hemorrhagic accidents in dental manipulations, extensive equimosis before minimal traumatism, big bruises, frequent epistaxis , etc. The clinical history must be completed by a careful physical examination of the patient who rejects the existence of signs corresponding to congenital affections or signs of affections that determine liver pathology (liver cirrhosis, vitamin C deficiency, etc.).

The signs of infection: fever, pain, inflammation, analytical parameters and the imaging technologies and procedures of drainages and obtaining of material adapted for later microbiological analyses were completing the diagnosis.

The diagnosis of a hematoma, infected or not infected, can prove difficult [7] because the only manifestation is local, insidious appearance, because it could confuse with tumor or other pathologies. The definitive diagnosis will be obtained by means of imaging explorations (TAC, Resonance, Ultrasound scan...) The imaging technologies cannot differ if a hematoma is infected or not, for what the sample for microbiological studies can result necessary majority of the occasions. The exploration by means of imaging technologies and microbiological sample by puncture aspiration can turn out to be besides diagnostic and therapeutic. Nevertheless in certain occasions the diagnosis by means of imaging explorations and the drainage with sample obtained by percutaneous route, can to be insufficient and there being needed more aggressive surgical procedures.

Microbiological Diagnosis

Since already it has been indicated, the obtaining of samples adapted by aspiration with needle or surgery is in the habit of contributing to a great extent to the etiologic diagnosis. They were taking blood cultures if bacteriemia is suspected. Besides the blood cultures the different samples can be inoculated in blood bottles (aerobic and anaerobic) to increase the diagnostic profitability. The transport of the sample to the laboratory of

Microbiology must be immediate and in suitable containers (aerobic and anaerobic).

For the high incident of anaerobic microorganisms [10,14,21,31,39,46, 53,94,115,122]they must be considered in the procedures of samples for microbiological studies and the procedures adapted for those microorganisms that are associated with infected hematomas and that do not grow in the ordinary cultures (for example *Mycoplasma hominis*).

The identification of the microorganisms is realized by means of direct antigen detection, when it is possible, by means of diverse methodologies. The molecular biology is diagnostic useful tools in the present and with a wide range of possibilities in the future [120]. In the majority of checked cases the hematoma cultures, the blood cultures and the culture from others samples have been diagnostic. In certain microorganism the serology can contribute to the diagnosis. The culture will contribute to the diagnosis and the antibiogram aide to the specific treatment.

9. Clinical Symptomatologie

The clinical expression of the entity changes according to the affected subjects, the affected organs and the responsible microorganisms. For it the clinical presentation will be very heterogeneous being able to appear of sharp, subsharp or chronic form. His diagnosis can turn out to be difficult for his scanty symptomatology, for his insidious appearance or for being confused with tumors or other pathologies. Fever, pain, and diverse symptomatology depending on the location can be present or no [123].

10. Differential Diagnosis

In the literature there are indexed erroneous diagnoses of piomiositis [92], appendicitis [35], tumors [15], necrotics tumors [1], aneurysms [79,101], subdural empyema, not infected hematomas [121] etc, entities that they must be considered before the suspicion of an infected or not infected hematoma. Spontaneous bled of an artery or of his branches and the consistent hematoma bruise and or the infection of this one is a rare entity that can get confused with muscular tear, piomiositis, gaseous gangrene or tromboflebitis. [121]

11. Treatment

Generally the drainage is in the habit of being necessary [106] due to the strong pain caused by the tisular compression. The percutaneous drainage [82] and or the aspiration together with the antibiotics, empirical first and specific after the antibiogram, can be decisive, except in the cases that compromise vital organs. In occasions they were turning out to be more aggressive necessary surgical technologies.

12. Evolution and Pronostic

The evolution of the infected hematomas is variable, being able to evolve towards the treatment or to turn into a chronic entity with a clinic silent that will delay the diagnosis and the treatment and with an unfavorable evolution. Bone hematomas are the most serious. Sometimes the existence of a membrane that delimits the hematoma avoids at first the spread of the infection. But the incident of systemic associate infections is high. [4,5,9] This way an infected hematoma can complicate with sepsis, bacteriemia, meningitis, osteomielitis [80], neuritis, epidural abscess, subdural empyema, pneumo-peritoneum [14], etc. Nevertheless great part of the infected published hematomas evolved favorably.

13. Conclusions

Hematomas can happen in any part of the body being capable of becoming infected immediately or of more late form for microorganisms of the endogenous flora and or exogenous microorganisms. His diagnosis and treatment must not delay by means of the technologies of image and the obtaining of samples adapted for cultures and or direct antigen detection were facilitating the diagnosis and the specific antibiotic treatment with the reduction of the morbidity-mortality.

The etiology more frequently associate has been *Escherichia coli* followed by anaerobic bacteria, *Staphylococcus aureus*, *Salmonella spp.* and *Mycoplasma hominis.*

In the checked bibliography scanty cases and series of few patients with infected hematomas are published, being able to be this one the first one or one of the scanty bibliographical reviews of infected hematomas in different anatomical locations published.

References

[1] Muccio CF, Leonini S, Esposito G, Cerase A. Pyogenic abscess from *Providencia stuartii* mimicking necrotic tumour at perfusion-weighted imaging. *Neurol Sci*, 2011 Oct;32(5):919-23.

[2] Kagami H, Muto J, Nakatukasa M, Inamasu J. Infected acute subdural hematoma associated with invasive pneumococcal disease. *Neurol Med Chir*, 2011;51(5):368-70.

[3] Koshiba H. Hematoma and abscess formation caused by *Mycoplasma hominis* following cesarean section. 27-year-old woman who developed abdominal wound hematoma and abscess after cesarean section. Int J Women's Health. 2011 Jan,17;3:15-8.

[4] Nakwan N, Wannaro J, Dissaneevate P, Kritsaneepaiboon S, Chokephaibulkit K. Septicemia, meningitis, and skull osteomyelitis complicating infected cephalhematoma caused by ESBL-producing *Escherichia coli. Southeast Asian J Trop Med Public Health* 2011 Jan;42(1):148-51.

[5] Bhooshan P, Shivaprakasha S, Dinesh KR, Kiran M, Karim P. Chronic subdural empyema and cranial vault osteomyelitis due to *Salmonella paratyphi A. Induian J Med Microbiol* 2010 Jan-Mar;28(1):60-2.

[6] Frye B, Prud'homme J, Daney B. Spontaneous bacterial seeding of a biceps hematoma.*Orthopedics* 2010 Nov, 2;33(11):848.

[7] Kruppa C, Goericke SL, Matheney T, Ozokyay L, Schildhauer TA, Muhr G, Dudda M. Blunt force injuries due to martial arts in children--a diagnostic problem? Delayed diagnosis of an infected hematoma. *Unfallchirurg* 2010 Oct;113(10):866-9.

[8] Iimura Y, Tsutsumi S, Mitome Y, Nonaka Y, Abe Y, Yasumoto Y, Ito M. Infantile chronic subdural hematoma infected by *Escherichia coli*-case report. *Neurol med Tokyo* 2010;50(6):482-4.

[9] Van Helleputte C, Dupont V, Barthels S, Aeby A. *Escherichia coli* meningitis and parietal osteomyelitis in an infant: a rare complication of cephalohematoma. *Rev Med Brux* 2010 Jan-Feb;31(1):57-9.

[10] López P, Belda S, García M, Royo G. Infection of a spontaneous muscular hematoma due to *Robinsoniella peoriensis*, in a patient with

alcoholic liver cirrhosis. Enferm Infecc Microbiol Clin. 2010 Oct;28(8):565-7.

[11] Brncić N, Mijandrusić-Sincić B, Perić R, Milić S, Gorup L, Mazur-Grbac M. A Splenic hematoma as a first manifestation of *Cytomegalovirus* infection. Coll Antropo 2010 Apr;34 Suppl 2:267-9.

[12] Tabarani CM, Bennett NJ, Kiska DL, Riddell SW, Botash AS, Domachowske JB. Empyema of preexisting subdural hemorrhage caused by a rare salmonella species after exposure to bearded dragons in a foster home. *J Pediatr* 2010 Febr;156(2):322-3. Hayakawa K, Oikawa A, Takeda N, Sasaki K, Hatakeyama S. Infected subdural haematoma due to *Salmonella enterica* serovar Typhimurium in an adult. *J med microb.* 2010 59(Pt 8):976-9.

[14] Cui H. Severe pneumoperitoneum caused by infected pelvic hematoma: report of a case and review of the literature. *Surg Infect* 2010 Feb;11(1):73-6.

[15] Kim CH, Kim JH, Lee HJ, Lee YS, Choi JH, Jung YK, Yeon JE, Byun KS.A case of liver abscess with subcapsular hematoma mimicking ruptured hepatic cholangiocarcinoma. *Korean J Gastroenterolog* 2009 Mar;53(3):202-5.

[16] Ahsan H, Ajmal F, Saleem MF, Sonawala AB. Cerebral fungal infection with mycotic aneurysm of basilar artery and subarachnoid haemorrhage. *Singapore Med J* 2009 Jan;50(1):e22-5.

[17] Weiss KJ, Edwards MS, Hay LM, Allen CH. *Escherichia coli-* infected cephalohematoma in an infant. *Clin Pediatr (Phila),* 2009 Sep;48(7):763-6..

[18] Tsubochi H, Sato N, Imai T. Chronic expanding hematoma with bronchopleural fistula and empyema space. *Ann Thorac Cardiovasc Surg* 2009 Jun;15(3):171-3.

[19] Hirshoren N, Gross M, Weinberger JM, Eliashar R. Retropharyngeal infected hematoma: a unique complication of nasogastric tube insertion. *J Trauma* 2009 Oct;67(4):891.

[20] Slap F, Jeurissen A, Van Havenbergh T, Deckers F, Mariën P, Van Mol C. Late onset subgaleal hemorrhage infection with *Streptococcus pneumoniae*?. *Europ J Pediatr* 2009 Jun;168(6):647-50.

[21] Kim JH, Lee CH, Hwang SH, Kang DH, Superimposed *Propionibacterium acnes* subdural empyema in a patient with chronic subdural hematoma. *J Corean Neurosug Soc.* 2009 Jan;45(1):53-6..

[22] Adem A, Olray E, Cosar M, Albayrak R. *Salmonella*-Infected Chronic Subdural Hematoma. *Turk J Med Sci* 2009; 39 (1): 139-142 (no Pubmed).

[23] Narita E, Maruya J, Nishimaki K, Heianna J, Miyauchi T, Nakahata J, Kitahara H, Minakawa T Case of infected subdural hematoma diagnosed by diffusion-weighted imaging. *Brain Nerve* 2009 Mar;61(3):319-23.

[24] Chau SY, Tiu SC. Spinal subdural haematoma: a rare complication of low-molecular-weight heparin therapy. Hong Kong Med J. 2008 Feb;14(1):64-6.

[25] Kanayama S, Ohnishi K, Yamaura T, Katayama M, Makino J, Takemura N, Hamabe Y. Case of bilateral subdural empyema complicating *Campylobacter fetus subspecies fetus* meningitis. *Brain Nerve* 2008 Jun;60(6):659-62.

[26] Hoshina T, Kusuhara K, Saito M, Mizoguchi M, Morioka T, Mizuno Y, Aoki T, Hara T. Infected subdural hematoma in an infant. *J Pn J Infect Dis* 2008 Sep;61(5):412-4.

[27] Abe M, Okada K, Matsumoto K. Iliopsoas hematoma consequent to prosthetic graft infection with methicillin-resistant *Staphylococcus aureus* in a hemodialysis patient. *Clin Nephro* 2008 Jun;69(6):465-8.

[28] Geldof K, Maleux G, Heye S, Van Cleynenbreugel B, Oyen R. Transcatheter embolization of an isolated lumbar arterial bleeding complicating radical nephrectomy for renal infarction with infected perirenal haematoma. *JBR BTR* 2008 Sep-Oct;91(5):203-5.

[29] Mesquita M, Damry N, Gazagnes MD Fatal cerebritis and brain abscesses following a nontraumatic subdural hematoma in a chronic hemodialyzed patient. *Hemodial Int* 2008 Oct;12(4):426-30.

[30] Jimeno A, García-Lechuz Moya JM, González E. Lesión cefálica de partes blandas en un niño de 9 meses. *Enferm Infecc Microbiol Clin* 2008;26(3):175-6 175.

[31] Mongil LL , Salvá P, García AB. Dolor abdominal y fiebre tras colangiopancreatografía retrógrada endoscópica (CPRE): hematoma hepático tras CPRE. *Rev Enf Ap Dig*. 2007;99:53-4 ISBN: 978-84-7989-625-6. No pubmed.

[32] Stief TW. Hemostasis and Infection/Inflammation, *Hemostasis Laboratory,* 2008 Vol 1, Issue 1, pp1-2.

[33] Godkar D, Anandacoomarswamy D, Bansal G, Patel R, Recco R. A rare case of infected splenic hematoma. *Am J Ther* 2007 Jul-Aug;14(4):411-3.

[34] Priego P, Rodríguez G, Mena A, Losa N, Aguilera A, Ramiro C, Lisa E, Conde S, Fresneda V. Hematoma subcapsular hepático tras CPRE *Rev. esp. enferm. dig.* 2007 Jan;99(1):53-4.

[35] Tranchart H, Fraleu Louër B. Infected rectus hematoma simulating an appendiceal abscess on CT scan. *J Chir Paris* 2007 Jul-Aug;144(4):357-8.

[36] Adamides AA, Goldschlager T, Tulloch SJ, McMahon JH. Pneumocephalus from gas-forming *Escherichia coli* subdural empyema. *Br J neurosurch* 2007 Jun;21(3):299-300.

[37] Le Roux PC. Subdural empyema caused by an unusual organism following intracranial haematoma. Childs Nerv Syst. 2007 Jul;23(7):825-7.

[38] Stief TW, Ijagha O, Weiste B, Herzum I, Renz H, Max M.Analysis of hemostasis alterations in sepsis. Source 2007 Mar;18(2):179-86.

[39] Pollack S, Kassis I, Soudack M, Sprecher H, Sujov P, Guilburd JN, Makhoul IR. Infected subgaleal hematoma in a neonate. *Pediatr Infec D* 2007 Aug;26(8):757-9.

[40] Otsuka T, Kato N, Kajiwara I, Tanaka T, Sawauchi S, Numoto RT, Murakami S, Abe T A case of infected subdural hematoma. *No shinkei Geka* 2007 Jan;35(1):59-63.

[41] Neto AC, da Silva MN, Mattos MH, Tristão RA, Wroclawski ER. Infected hepatic hematoma after renal extracorporeal shock wave lithotripsy. *Clinics Sao Paolo* 2006 Jun;61(3):275-6.

[42] Chen MH, Yang JC, Huang JS, Chen MH. MRI features of an infected cephalohaematoma in a neonate. *J Clin Neurosci* 2006 oct:13(8):849-52.

[43] Bomke AK, Feyerherd P, Podbielski A. Postoperative infection of an epigastric hematoma caused by Aeromonas veronii biovar sobria *Dtsch Med Wochenschr* 2006 Nov 24;131(47):2649-52.

[44] Sato K, Yamada M, Shimzu S, Utsuki S, Konno S, Fujii K, Kan S. Infected and calcified chronic subdural hematoma presenting an attitude of acute hematoma on MRI: case report. *No Shinkei Geka* 2005 Aug;33(8):805-8.

[45] van den Berge M, de Marie S, Kuipers T, Jansz AR, Bravenboer B. Psoas abscess: report of a series and review of the literature. *Neth J Med.*2005 Nov;63(10):413-6.

[46] Brook I. Infected neonatal cephalohematomas caused by anaerobic bacteria. *J Perinat Med.* 2005;33(3):255-8..

[47] Chang HY, Chiu NC, Huang FY, Kao HA, Hsu CH, Hung HY Infected cephalohematoma of newborns: experience in a medical center in Taiwan. *Pediatr Int.* 2005 Jun;47(3):274-7.

[48] Game X, Mouzin M, Vaessen C, Malavaud B, Sarramon JP, Rischmann P. Obturator infected hematoma and urethral erosion following transobturator tape implantation. *Journal Urol.* 2004;171(4):1629.

[49] Oshita J, Kiya K, Satoh H, Mizoue T, Nabika S, Araki H Four cases of the infectious cerebral aneurysms. *No Shinkei Geka* 2004 Dec;32(12):1263-8.

[50] Eggink BH, Richardson CJ, Rowen JL. Gardnerella vaginalis-infected scalp hematoma associated with electronic fetal monitoring. *Pediatr Infec J* 2004 Mar;23(3):276-8.

[51] Arena F, Romeo C, Manganaro A, Centorrino A, Basile M, Arena S, Romeo G. Bilateral neonatal adrenal abscess. Report of two cases and review of the literature *Pediatr Med Chir* 2003 May-Jun;25(3):185-9.

[52] Yamakawa H, Hattori T, Tanigawara T, Enomoto Y, Ohkuma A. Ruptured infectious aneurysm of the distal middle cerebral artery manifesting as intracerebral hemorrhage and acute subdural hematoma--case report. *Neurol Med Chirug*, 2003 Nov;43(11):541-5.

[53] Castiglioni B, Gautam A, Citron DM, Pasculle W, Goldstein EJ, Strollo D, Jordan M, Kusne S. *Clostridium innocuum* bacteremia secondary to infected hematoma with gas formation in a kidney transplant recipient. *Tansplant Infect dis* 2003 Dec;5(4):199-202.

[54] Douglas MW. Mycoplasma hominis infection of a subdural haematoma in the peripartum period. Pathology. 2003 Oct;35(5):452-4.

[55] Yanagihara C, Wada Y, Nishimura Y. Infectious endocarditis associated with subarachnoid hemorrhage, subdural hematoma and multiple brain abscesses. *Intern med* 2003 Dec;42(12):1244-7.

[56] Neuman M. Infected hematoma following tension-free vaginal tape implantation. *J urol* 2002 Dec;168(6):2549.

[57] Vaidyanathan S, Soni BM, Hughes PL, Singh G, Watt JW, Oo T, Sett P. How should an infected perinephric haematoma be drained in a tetraplegic patient with baclofen pump implanted in the abdominal wall? - A case report. *BMC Urol* 2002 Sep 10;2:9.

[58] Fan HC, Hua YM, Juan CJ, Fang YM, Cheng SN, Wang CC. Infected cephalohematoma associated with sepsis and scalp cellulitis: a case report. *J Microbiol Immunol Infect* 2002 Jun;35(2):125-8.

[59] Honda M, Tanaka K, Tanaka S, Nakayama T, Kaneko M, Ozawa T , A case of infected subdural hematoma following chronic subdural hematoma irrigation. *No To Shinkei Article* 2002 Aug;54(8):703-6.

[60] Ishii N, Hirano K, Mouri Y, Imamura K, Kamata M, Watanabe A, Suzuki Y, Ishii R, A case of infected subdural hematoma due to *Campyrobacter fetus*. *No shinkei geka* 2001 Mar;29(3):265-9.

[61] Triki A, Essid I, Trabelsi S, Rhouma M, Gara MF, Mestiri T, Bouhaja B, Ben Ammar MS. Subcapsular liver hematoma. Two case reports and review of the Literature. Jan; *Tunis Med* 2001 79(1):58-61.

[62] Montravers P, Villamizar J, Sansom A, Barsam E, Agaesse V, Abourachid H, Moubarak M. Superinfection of posttraumatic retroperitoneal hematoma secondary to ascending urinary tract infection. *J Trauma* 2001 May;50(5):931-3.

[63] Goodwin MD, Persing JA, Duncan CC, Shin JH. Spontaneously infected cephalohematoma: case report and review of the literature. discussion. *J craneofac cirug* 2000 Jul;11(4):371-5;.

[64] Legg JM, Titus TT. Hematoma infection with *Mycoplasma hominis* following transplant nephrectomy. Clin Microbiol Infect 2000 Nov;6(11):619-21.

[65] Escamilla F, Fernández MD, Espigares A, Arnal C, Ortega A, García T.Subdural empyema due to *Mycoplasma hominis* following epidural anesthesia. *Rev neurol* 2000 Feb 16-29;30(4):326-8.

[66] Kao HC, Huang YC, Lin TY. Infected cephalohematoma associated with sepsis and skull osteomyelitis: report of one case. *Am J Perinatol* 1999;16(9):459-62.

[67] Sawauchi S, Saguchi T, Miyazaki Y, Ikeuchi S, Ogawa T, Yuhki K, Abe T. Infected subdural hematoma. *J Clin Neurosci* 1998 Apr;5(2):233-7.

[68] Kawamoto S, Nagata K, Mochizuki Y, Hara T, Abe T, Sashida J. Subdural empyema caused by hematogenous dissemination from an abscess in muslo thigh to a preexisting chronic subdural hematoma--case report. *Neurol med chir Tokyo* 1998 Nov;38(11):743-5.

[69] Mori S, Imaizumi M, Takeuchi M, Takeuchi S, Hiramatsu Y, Yoshioka H, Watanabe H, Iwashita T. A case of intrathoracic chronic expanding hematoma. *Kyobu Geka* 1998 Feb;51(2):161-3.

[70] Aoki N, Sakai T, Oikawa A, Takizawa T, Shishido T. Infected subdural effusion associated with resolving subdural hematoma--case report. *Neurol Med Chirug* 1997 Aug;37(8):637-9.

[71] Kamiński Z, Lukasik M. Mediastinal abscesses and empyema of the pleural cavity after iatrogenic fracture of the sternum. *Pol Merkur Lekarski* 1997 Dec;3(18):279-80.

[72] Duffner F, Brandner S, Opitz H, Klier R, Grote EH. Primary *Candida albicans* empyema associated with epidural hematomas in craniocervical junction. *Clin neuropathol* 1997 May-Jun;16(3):143-6.

[73] Cerwenka H, Werkgartner G, Bacher H, el-Shabrawi A, Mischinger HJ. Intrahepatic hematoma with secondary Salmonella infection via biliary fistula. *Hepatogastroenterlogy.*1997 Mar-Apr;44(14):529-32.

[74] Yamasaki F, Kodama Y, Hotta T, Taniguchi E, Hashizume A, Kajiwara Y, Yamane T. A case of infected subdural hematoma complicating chronic subdural hematoma in a healthy adult man. *No To shinkeii* 1997 Jan;49(1):81-4.

[75] Lindberg JA, Mouritsen EA. Gluteal hematoma infected with multiresistant *Salmonella typhi*. *Ugeskr Laeger* 1997 Dec 29;160(1):54-5.

[76] Hirano A, Takamura T, Murayama N, Ohyama K, Matsumura S, Niwa J. Subdural abscess following chronic subdural hematoma]. *No shinkei geka*. 1995 Jul;23(7):643-6.

[77] Bakker S, Kluytmans J, den Hollander JC, Lie ST. Subdural empyema caused by *Escherichia coli*: hematogenous dissemination to a preexisting chronic subdural hematoma. *Clin infec diseas* 1995 Aug;21(2):458-9.

[78] Haight DO, Toney JF, Greene JN, Sandin RL, Vincent AL. Liver abscess following blunt trauma: a case report and review of the literature. *Shout Med J* 1994 Aug;87(8):811-3.

[79] Berry MC, Van Schil PE, Vanmaele RG, De Vries DP. Infected false aneurysm after puncture of an aneurysm of the deep femoral artery. *Europ J Vasc Cir*, 1994 May;8(3):372-4.

[80] Blom NA, Vreede WB. Infected cephalhematomas associated with osteomyelitis, sepsis and meningitis. *Pediatr Infect dis* 1993 Dec;12(12):1015-7.

[81] Haller M, Forst H, Ruckdeschel G, Pratschke E. Mycoplasma hominis in liver transplantation. *Surgery* 1993 Mar;113(3):359-60.

[82] García-Vila J, Sáiz-Pachés V, Doménech-Iglesias MA, González-Añon M, Selfa-Moreno S, Esteban-Ricós MJ, Montes-Benito H. Infected intraabdominal hematomas: percutaneous drainage. *Abdmon Imagin* 1993 Fall;18(4):313-7.

[83] Fusato G, Vidali M, Zuccarotto D, Rodighiero D. Hematomas of the abdominal rectus muscle. *Minerva Chir* 1993 Feb;48(3-4):107-13.

[84] Orange GV, Jones M, Henderson IS. Wound and perinephric haematomata infection with *Mycoplasma hominis* in a renal transplant recipient. Nephrol Dial Transplant. 1993;8(12):1395-6.

[85] Andersen E, Skadberg JE. Abdominal wall hematoma.Tidsskr Nor Laegeforen. *Kirurgisk avdeling* 1992 Aug 20;112(19):2529-30.

[86] Bartels RH, de Jong TR, Grotenhuis JA Spinal subdural abscess. Case report. *J Neurosurch* 1992 Feb;76(2):307-11.

[87] Jacobs F, Van de Stadt J, Gelin M, Nonhoff C, Gay F, Adler M, Thys JP. *Mycoplasma hominis* infection of perihepatic hematomas in a liver transplant recipient. *Surgery*.1992 Jan;111(1):98-100.

[88] Redondo Granado MJ. Salmonella C1 splenic abscess in a hematoma An Esp Pediatr. An Esp Pediatr 1992 Jan;36(1):67-8.

[89] Weigel M, Friese K, Schmitt W, Strittmatter HJ, Melchert F. Infected chorionic hematoma as a cause of infection in the 2nd trimester. *Geburtshilfe Frauenheilkd* 1992 Dec;52(12):780-2.

[90] Lizardo-Barahona JR, Nieto-Zermeño J, Bracho-Blanchet E. Adrenal abscess in the newborn: a case report and review of the literature. *Bol Med* 1990 Jun;47(6):401-4.

[91] Klein JH. Muscular hematomas: diagnosis and management. *J Manipulative Physiol Ther.* 1990 Feb;13(2):96-100.

[92] Back SA, O'Neill T, Fishbein G, Gwinup G, case of *group B streptococcal* pyomyositis. *Rev infect dis.*1990 Sep-Oct;12(5):784-7.

[93] Meignier M, Renaud P, Robert R, Roze JC, Rigal E, Mouzard A. Cephalhematoma infection in neonatal septicemia. *Pediatrie* 1989;44(1):27-9.

[94] Suhr GM, Green AE Jr. Rectus abdominis sheath hematoma as a complication of tetanus. Diagnosis by computed tomography scanning. *Clin imaging* 1989 Mar;13(1):82-6.

[95] Itoh S, Hara M, Asoh Y, Yokoyama H, Ogashiwa M, Takeuchi K.Infected chronic subdural hematoma due to an ethmoiditis; a case report. *Rinsho Hoshasen* 1989 Feb;34(2):257-60.

[96] Kailath EJ, Hrdy DB. Hematoma infected with *Mycoplasma hominis. Sex Transm Dis* 1988 Apr-Jun;15(2):114-5.

[97] Alembik Y, Donato L, Roy C, Stoll C. Radiologic case of the month. Pneumatocele on infected intrapulmonary hematoma. *Arch Franch Pediatrie Alembyk Y Pediatrie* 1988 Oct;45(8):573-4.

[98] Vogelzang RL, Tobin RS, Burstein S, Anschuetz SL, Marzano M, Kozlowski JM. Transcatheter intracavitary fibrinolysis of infected extravascular hematomas. *AJT Am J Roentgenol* 1987 Feb;148(2):378-80.

[99] Morduchowicz G, Rabinovitz M, Neuman M, Pitlik S. Infected renal hematoma complicating anticoagulant therapy. *Isr J Med Sci* 1987 Mar;23(3):202-4.

[100] Tokunaga Y, Inoue M, Ishizaka H, Koga H, Kawano T, Mori K. Encapsulated subdural empyema--a case report with special reference to CT findings and operative indications. *No shinkei geka* 1985 Apr;13(4):433-6.

[101] Gubko AA. Infected false aneurysm of the deep femoral artery. *Khirurgia Mosk.*1985 Dec;(12):115-6.

[102] Handrick W, Hückel D, Spencker FB, Kühnert C. Infected scalp hematoma, *Zentralbl Gynakol* 1983;105(15):1011-3.

[103] Boles JM, Vallee B, Lejeune B, Le Cam B, Brousse A, Garre M, Chastel C. *Salmonella*-infected subdural haematoma. J Infect. 1983 Jul;7(1):67-71.

[104] Loup J. Infected retroperitoneal traumatic hematoma. *Sem Hop* 1983 Jun 9;59(23):1761-2.

[105] Khan MI, Chan R. *Pasteurella multocida* subdural empyema: a case report. *Can J Neurol* 1981 May;8(2):163-5..

[106] Karlson KB, Martin EC, Fankuchen EI, Mattern RF, Cooperman AM, Rose EA, Gold RP, Casarella WJ. Non-surgical drainage of intra-abdominal and mediastinal abscesses: a report of twelve cases. *Cardiocasc Intervent Radiol* 1981;4(3):170-6.

[107] Burke DS, Madoff S. Infection of a traumatic pelvic hematoma with *Mycoplasma hominis*. Sex Transm Dis. 1978 Apr-Jun;5(2):65-7.

[108] Gleicher N, Gergely ZR, Deppe G. An infected ovarian hematoma as the presenting symptom of systemic lupus erythematosus. *J Reprod Med* 1978 Oct;21(4):223-7.

[109] Diwan N, Sharma KB. Isolation of *Salmonella typhimurium* from cephalhematoma and osteomyelitis.Indian J Med Res.1978 Jan;67:27-9.

[110] Vetrovec GW, Warner JF. Infected subdural hematoma: three case reports involving gram-negative organisms. Am J Med Sci. 1975 Jan-Feb;269(1):113-5.

[111] Lerner PI, Golden PF, Jane JA. *Salmonella*-infected subdural hematoma.Pediatrics. 1972 Jan;49(1):127-8.

[112] Chan MC, Boon WH Infected cephalhaematoma. *J Singapore Ped Soc.*1972 Apr;14(1):57-60.

[113] Lee Y, Berg RB Cephalhematoma infected with *Bacteroides. Am J Dis Child* 1971 Jan;121(1):77-8..

[114] Ewbank RL, DHOM H.,Unusual infected hematoma: report of case. *Deutsche Zahnarztl Z* 1969 Oct;79(4):898-900.

[115] Levy HL, O'Connor JF, Ingall D. Bacteremia, infected cephalhematoma, and osteomyelitis of the skull in a newborn. *Am J Dis Child* 1967 Dec;114(6):649-51.

[116] Geetter DM, Flanigan S. Infected subdural hematoma. *Conn med* 1967 Feb;31(2):115-8.

[117] DHOM H. Neuritis of the nervus infraorbitalis caused by an infected hematoma after tuberal anesthesia. *Deutsche Zahnarztl. Z.*1954 Oct 1;9(19):1114-6.

[118] Guilhem P, Pontonnier A, Monrozies M. Two cases of infected hematoma of the broad ligament after low transverse cesarean section. *Bull Fed Soc Gynecol Obstet Lang Fr* 1953;5(2):248-9.

[119] KLOS HJ. Subdural empyema probably secondary to infected chronic subdural hematoma; case report. *Harper Hosp Bull.*1949 May-Jun;7(3):232-5.

[120] Eser O, Cosar M, Aslan A, Koken R, Aktepe F, Eser B. Intracerebral hematoma complicated with brain abscess in an infant. Case report.*Neurol Med Chir.* 2008 Apr;48(4):176-8.

[121] Karagol BS, Zencıroglu A, Kundak AA, Okumus N, Aydin M, Uner C. A linear fracture and meningitis associated with non-infected cephalohematoma in a neonate. *Neuropediatrics.* 2010 Dec;41(6):276-8.

[122] Murray PR, Baron EJ, Jorgensen JH, Landry ML, Pfaller MA, *Manual of Clinical Microbiology*, Washinghton DC ASM Press, 9thEdition, 2007.

[123] Mandell BD, *Principles and Practice of Infectious Diseases,* Chrichill Livingstone, 6thEdition, 2009.

In: Hematomas: Types, Treatments … ISBN: 978-1-61942-385-5
Editors: M.F.G.Salazar…pp. 121-141

Chapter IV

Pelvic Hematomas: Types and Management

Maria Consuelo Calomarde, Ignacio Zapardiel* and Javier De Santiago
Obstetrics and Gynecology Department.
La Paz University Hospital. Madrid. Spain

Abstract

Pelvic hematomas are collections of blood located in the pelvic peritoneal space, as a result of bleeding lacerations after operative deliveries or during gynecologic surgery. In the pelvic abdominal cavity, hematomas may take place in the uterovesical space, rectouterine pouch (Douglas space) or in **paravesical,** parametrial, paracervical, paravaginal or pararectal areas.

Concerning its etiology, it could be classified in obstetrical, gynecological and others causes. The most frequent obstetrical cause are puerperal hematomas that occur in 1:300 to 1:1500 deliveries and they are a potentially life-threatening complication of childbirth. The most common locations are the vulva, vaginal/paravaginal area and retroperitoneum due to an injury of uterine artery, and most rarely of the hypogastric artery during hysterotomy.

* Email: ignaciozapardiel@hotmail.com

Regarding gynecological causes, surgical procedures may lead to the injury of paracervical and paravaginal vessels, ovarian vessels, uterine artery or rarely external or internal iliac vessels with major blood loss.

Other causes of pelvic hematoma include trauma, anticoagulating drugs and coagulation disease, ruptured ectopic pregnancy and ruptured of an aneurysm in the abdominopelvic vasculature.

Symptoms usually develop in the first 24 hours after delivery or surgery and vary depending on the location of the hematoma. Commonly they are associated with pain and effects caused by the hypovolemia. The three primary approaches for managing pelvic hematomas are: conservative management with observation, surgical intervention and selective arterial embolization. Evaluation of a patient with suspected postoperative or puerperal bleeding includes physical examination and assessment of vital signs and urine output. Patients who are conservatively managed should be observed closely. Surgical intervention must be carried out if growing hematoma is evidenced on physical examination or imaging studies, or hematocrite value decrease is observed.

General Aspects and Pelvic Anatomy

Pelvic hematomas are collections of blood located in the pelvic peritoneal space, as a result of bleeding lacerations after operative deliveries or during gynecologic surgery. The uterus, vagina and vulva have rich vascular supplies that are at risk of trauma in many situations and it may result in formation of an hematoma.

The pelvic extraperitoneal cavity is a part of the retroperitoneal space extending from the pubic symphysis to the sacrum. Connective-tissue septa separate pelvic extraperitoneal organs, providing mechanical support and a path for vascular and lymphatic vessels and nerves, and they serve as natural barriers to the spread of infection, cancer and hematomas.

The cervix and vagina receive their blood supply from several sources, with the largest blood vessels lying on the lateral wall. Laceration of the vaginal wall can cause significant hemorrhage if these arteries are damaged, and internal hematomas can form between the vagina and the elevator ani muscle, inferior to the cardinal ligament. Paravaginal hematomas can be classified into supraelevator and infraelevator hematomas .

Supraelevator hematomas extend superiorly and involve the broad ligament, whereas infraelevator hematomas extend to the vulva, perineum, and ischiorectal fossa. The ischiorectal fossa does not connect with the extraperitoneal space.

Because of the uterine enlargement in pregnant women, the broad ligament extends quite superiorly and forms a large potential space between the anterior and posterior layers, into which a large amount of blood can seep.

Pelvic hematomas can extend to the perivesical, vesicovaginal, or rectovaginal spaces.

The vesicovaginal (vesicocervical) fascia, the rectovaginal septum, or the umbilicovesical fascia acted as a barrier, whereas the paravesical and pararectal spaces are composed of fat and loose connective tissue, and these spaces communicate with each other.

The pelvis is richly supplied by blood, and there are many anastomoses present from branches of the internal iliac artery that is a major branch of the distal abdominal aorta. The aorta bifurcates at the level of L4 into right and left common iliac arteries. These vessels course along the pelvic sidewall and exit the pelvis via the iliac fossa. The common iliac artery bifurcates into the external and the internal iliac arteries. The internal iliac artery dives deep into the pelvis and gives rise to branches which supply the reproductive tract. These include: obturator artery, umbilical artery, uterine-vaginal artery, superior and inferior vesical arteries.

The upper vagina is supplied by the vaginal branch of the uterine artery. After this branch to the coronary artery of the cervix, the vaginal artery supplies the anterior vagina and lower two-thirds of the urethra with multiple branches, along with anastomoses from the azygos artery (which is a continuation of the coronary artery). Eventually, this anastomoses to the urethral branch of the clitoral artery. The posterior vaginal wall is supplied by branches of the middle and inferior hemorrhoidal arteries. These branches then anastomose on the perineum to the superficial and deep transverse perineal arteries as Fadi M and Sreedhar G published.

Blood is supplied to the uterus primarily by the uterine artery which is a terminal branch of the internal iliac artery. It ascends along the lateral aspect of the uterus on either side giving off branches which penetrate into the myometrium.

The primary source of blood to the ovary is provided by the ovarian artery. These vessels, frequently called gonadal arteries, are usually originated from the abdominal aorta, it may also arise from the renal artery. It courses through folds of the suspensory ligaments and pierces the ovary at its hilus. Branches radiate circumferentially from the hilus into the ovarian parenchyma.

Etiology and Management

Concerning the etiology of pelvic hematomas, it could be classified in obstetrical, gynecological and others causes.

A. Obstetrical Causes

In spite of using a precise obstetrical technique, the forces of labor and expulsion of the fetus will sometimes result in lacerations of the lower genital tract. During pregnancy the uterus, vagina and vulva have rich vascular supplies that are at risk of trauma during delivery, and trauma may result in formation of an hematoma. The incidence of puerperal hematomas is not constant in the literature, ranging from approximately 1:300 to 1:1500 deliveries This range is in part due to the lack of a standard definition of a puerperal hematoma. Rarely, are a potentially life-threatening complication of childbirth.

Risk factors for injuring the pelvic vasculature and hematoma formation include operative deliveries or episiotomy, however, a hematoma may also result from injury to a blood vessel in the absence of laceration of the surrounding tissue. Also women at increased risk of developing puerperal hematomas include those who are nulliparous or who have infant over 4.000 grams, preeclampsia, prolonged second stage of labor, delivery of multiples, vulvar varicosities or clotting disorders.

Hematomas are most often classified according to location, which is defined by visualization, examination and palpation. Using this approach, puerperal hematomas have been defined as vulvar, vaginal/paravaginal, and retroperitoneal.

a) Vulvar hematomas, which are infralevator in location, can be further defined by the anterior triangle or posterior triangle. Most vulvar hematomas result from injuries to branches of the pudendal artery (inferior rectal, perineal, posterior labial, and urethral arteries; the artery of the vestibule; and the deep and dorsal arteries of the clitoris) that occur during episiotomy or from perineal lacerations. The superficial compartment of the anterior triangle, bleeding is confined by the perineal membrane preventing extension into the ischiorrectal fossa, superiorly by the levator ani, and limited from spread onto the thigh by Colles' fascia and the fascia lata. The central tendon of the perineum, or perineal body, prevents these hematomas from spreading beyond midline. Bleeding in the posterior triangle is limited by the anal fascia; however, because the perineal membrane does not extend to this area around the rectum, bleeding can dissect into ischiorectal fossa.

As a result, bleeding is directed towards the skin where the loose subcutaneous tissues afford little resistance to hematoma formation. Necrosis caused by pressure and rupture of the tissue surrounding the hematoma may lead to external hemorrhage.

b) Vaginal/paravaginal hematomas occur due to bleeding from the descending branches of uterine artery, mainly the descending branch. They are commonly associated with forceps delivery, but may also occur during spontaneous delivery.

In contrast to the vulva, vessels in the vagina are surrounded by soft tissue and do not lie in the superficial fascia; therefore, trauma to these vessels can lead to a large accumulation of blood in the paravaginal space or ischiorectal fossa. Vulvovaginal hematomas may involve either side of the levator plate, but if there is bleeding in the upper two-thirds of the vagina, this represents supralevator hematomas, which usually dissect paravaginally and may have significant extension into the retroperitoneal space. This extension and dissection into the retroperitoneum may occur and form a palpable tumor above Poupart's ligament. Dissection may also extend cephalad, potentially reaching the lower margin of the diaphragm.

c) Retroperitoneal hematomas, compared to vulvar and vaginal/paravaginal hematomas, are a rare complication of childbirth. During peripartum period, retroperitoneal hematomas occur secondary to laceration of branches of the uterine artery and/or vessels of the broad ligament, and are the least common hematoma encountered with an estimated incidence of 1:3500 to 1:20.000.

Although these usually occur following cesarean section (unrecognized extensions into the broad ligament), they can also occur because of uterine scar dehiscence during the first or second stage of labor or from uterine rupture and extension of a paravaginal hematoma. The resulting hemorrhage can be quite severe and lead to immediate hemodynamic instability.

Diagnosis

The diagnosis of most puerperal hematomas is based on the presence of characteristic symptoms and findings on physical examination. Symptoms usually develop in the first 24 hours after delivery.

The patient may require analgesia in order to allow a thorough examination. It can be associated with pain and proportionally to the size of the injury due to the sensitivity of this area.

The clinical presentation of the pelvic hematomas can be useful in defining the location of the bleeding vessel. Although small hematomas may be asymptomatic, majority are associated with pain and mass effect. A large mass may displace the vagina or rectum and hemodynamic instability may result from continued significant bleeding.

Vulvar hematomas usually present with rapid development of painful, tense and compressible mass covered by skin with purplish discoloration, which is usually greater than anticipated from a routine episiotomy. A vulvar hematoma may be an extension of a vaginal hematoma that has dissected through loose subcutaneous tissue into the vulva.

Patients with vaginal hematomas, or vulvovaginal hematomas involving the ischiorectal fossa, will present pain, and the physical examination will demonstrate a mass that causes rectal pressure; however , hemodynamic instability due to bleeding into the ischiorectal fossa and paravaginal space may be the first symptom of a vaginal hematoma, and it can result in hypovolemic shock. On physical examination, a large mass protruding into the vagina is usually obvious.

Retroperitoneal hematomas extending between the folds of the broad ligament may be asymptomatic initially. Supralevator and retroperitoneal hematomas usually present with hemodynamic instability due to the significant amount of blood that can accumulate in the retroperitoneal space. Patients with a retroperitoneal hematoma usually do not present with pain unless the hematoma is associated with trauma. Palpation of an abdominal mass or fever can also be signs of a retroperitoneal hematoma.

Diagnostic imaging in suspected vulvar or vaginal hematomas is rarely necessary. However, it may be useful to aid in determining the size and precise location of the hematoma and whether it is expanding, it also may be used to identify nonpalpable hematomas in puerperal women with pain or pressure suggestive of a hematoma, particularly retroperitoneal hematomas. Puerperal hematomas should be suspected in all postpartum patients who demonstrate signs of acute blood loss or hypovolemia, such as unexplained tachycardia or decreased urine output. As with all cases of hemorrhage (both obstetrical and non- obstetrical) imaging studies should not delay appropriate intervention to stabilize the patient and control bleeding if the patient is hemodynamically unstable.

When imaging is indicated, we suggest sonography for initial evaluation, followed by computed tomography if there is a suspicion for a retroperitoneal hematoma that cannot be visualized on ultrasound. Since the purpose of imaging is to help identify the location and size of the hematoma and not to identify a bleeding vessel, injection of contrast is not necessary. Information obtained from diagnostic imaging can facilitate the decision-making process regarding conservative versus interventional management and the appropriate interventional technique. Gemer et al evaluated the incidence of ultrasonographically-diagnosed postcesarean hematomas and correlate their presence with febrile morbidity, they concluded that a subfascial hematoma has the potential for significant spread, and its volume is difficult to estimate. In addition, its presence should be specifically sought when evaluating a febrile postcesarean patient.

Management

Recognition of a hematoma and prompt stabilization of the patient are the initial steps in the management of all hematomas. Thorough physical examination of the abdomen, vulva, vagina and rectum (including visual inspection of the external genitalia, vagina, and cervix) should be performed to determine the location and size of the hematoma.

Hemodynamically stable patients almost always have venous bleeding; arterial bleeding invariably results in hemodynamic instability. If the patient is hemodynamically stable, we place a large- bore intravenous lines and begin volume resuscitation with crystalloid and blood products as clinically indicated to stabilize the patient as we make preparations for surgical intervention or embolization via interventional radiology. We also order a complete blood count, fibrinogen level, prothrombin time, and partial thromboplastin time to determine baseline levels and whether a bleeding diathesis is present. The repair of large and expanding puerperal hematomas almost always requires regional or general anesthesia to control pain. Antibiotics should be generally administered to patients undergoing surgical intervention.

The three primary approaches for managing puerperal hematomas are conservative management with observation and supportive care, surgical intervention, and selective arterial embolization. The literature is no conclusive regarding the benefits of conservative treatment versus surgical intervention.

Patients who are conservatively managed should be observed closely. It is essential to monitor for signs of hypovolemia, suggestive of persistent or severe hemorrhage. Most patients will require administration of analgesia and these medications need to be taken into account when assessing overall status. It is important to keep in mind the usual hemodynamic changes that occur in the postpartum period. Patients can experience significant blood loss without changes in blood pressure. Laboratory studies may be needed every four to six hours, depending on the clinical presentation. Imaging modalities, such as ultrasound, are performed serially, as needed, to determine if there is an expansion of the hematoma.

Small vulvar hematomas will often solve with conservative management. Ice packs applied to the perineum for the first 24 hours help to minimize swelling, and analgesia should be administered to manage the pain. Large vulvar hematomas often interfere with urination so a Foley catheter should be placed upon initial evaluation. There are no proven criteria that can be used to select vulva hematomas likely to have a better outcome with surgical intervention rather than supportive care. Some authors suggested surgical intervention when the patient have significant pain or expansion of the hematoma, or if the hematoma is > 5 cm or an estimated volume > 200 ml as Zahn CM et al published. Another group advised surgical intervention if the product of the longitudinal dimension and transverse dimension is ≥ 15 cm^2. There is a general consensus that prompt surgical intervention is necessary if there is expansion of the hematoma on physical examination or imaging studies, or falling hematocrit, some persistent hemorrhage can lead to hemodynamic instability or put the tissue at risk of necrosis. The skin over the hematoma is incised and the clot evacuated. Detectable bleeding points should be legated if identified; however, in most cases, the lacerated vessel cannot be identified. Bleeding leading to a vulvar hematoma is often venous and from multiple sites. The space created by the hematoma is reapproximated using interrupted or figure-of-eight stitches of a fine, rapidly absorbable, synthetic suture such as monocryl or polyglactin 910.

The approach to vaginal hematomas is similar than for vulvar hematomas. Vaginal hematomas larger than approximately 4 cm may need to be evacuated. Patients conservatively managed are followed with as described above . If surgical intervention is required, good surgical exposure is important, as these hematomas are less accessible than vulvar hematomas. Evacuation usually needs to be done under general or regional anesthesia in an operating room, where good lighting, appropriate surgical instruments and a surgical assistant is available.

If the hematoma is at the site of a laceration that has been repaired, should be the hematoma cavity should be inspected to determine the extent of the injury and identify bleeding vesels, which are individually ligated. Most clinicians close the defect in layers using a fine, rapidly absorbable synthetic suture. The proximity of the bladder anteriorly, small bowel and rectum posteriorly, and the ureters and uterine vessels deep in the lateral vaginal fornices are important to consider when closing the defect, as they can be included in placement of large deep sutures. If electrocautery is used to achieve hemostasis, it is important to avoid deep or widespread thermal injury because of the vagina's proximity to the bowel and bladder, as well as risk of infection in the resulting necrotic tissue. We close the vaginal epithelium with a running locked absorbable suture. The anchoring stitch is placed above the apex of laceration and each stitch extends to the base of the opening to avoid creating pockets for hematoma/seroma formation.

Vaginal packing with gauze or a balloon for 12 or 24 hours may aid in tamponade. A Foley catheter may be necessary to drain the bladder in the presence of a vaginal pack or significant edema.

There are no randomized clinical trials comparing surgical approach versus angiographic treatment for the management of retroperitoneal hematomas, so their management is more controversial. Both have been advocated, but it is clear that blood replacement therapy is a hallmark of this type of hematoma. The retroperitoneal space is a large cavity, many patients with a retroperitoneal hematoma require either surgical or angiographic intervention. However, since it is a confined space, conservative management may be enough because the hematoma tamponades slowly bleeding vessels.

- ✓ Surgery – Laparotomy is required in virtually all cases of puerperal retroperitoneal bleeding. Most of these patients are hemodynamically unstable and most cases are associated with uterine rupture or cesarean delivery, both of which require laparotomy to repair the uterus. The incidence of uterine rupture varies in the literature but is estimated close to 0'1%. Numerous risk factors have been linked to uterine rupture, including prior cesarean delivery, uterine surgery, congenital uterine malformations, agents used for induction of labor and termination of pregnancy, and trauma. The American College of Obstetricians and Gynecologists (ACOG) recognizes that labor is a safe and reasonable management option for certain patients, and it may help limit the continued rise in cesarean section rates. However, ACOG directs that vaginal delivery following cesarean section should be limited to patients with one previous low-transverse cesarean delivery, with clinically adequate pelvis and no other uterine scars or history of prior rupture.

- ✓ Hemostasis can be achieved after opening the retroperitoneal space by identifying and ligating the lacerated blood vessel or by ligating the hypogastric artery. As with the other types of puerperal hematomas, identification of the bleeding vessel may be difficult. Ligation of the ipsilateral hypogastric artery usually stops the bleeding and avoids the delay associated to the searching for the bleeding origin. If bleeding does not respond to ipsilateral hypogastric artery ligation, then bilateral hypogastric artery ligation should be performed. Although hypogastric artery ligation reduces pelvic blood flow by about one-half, it has a greater impact on pulse pressure distal to the ligation (85 percent reduction), reducing pulse pressures to that of the venous circuit which promotes hemostasis. The procedure will be described forwards in gynecologic surgery. Selective uterine or hypogastric (internal iliac) artery ligation and mass uterine artery are surgical options for avoiding hysterectomy in intractable postpartum hemorrhage. The techniques, which all require laparotomy, were described back in 1950s. In one of the largest retrospective series on the uterine artery ligation covering 30 years which was published by O'Leary in 1995 who reported only ten failures in 265 patients. However, no literature is available on the use of the vaginal route for uterine artery lagation in intractable obstetric hemorrhage, although the technique is simple, highly effective, and avoids laparotomy. Gundula Hebisch et al conclude in their study that the vaginal route offers a novel, simple, effective, and minimally invasive technique for treating intractrable puerperal hemorrhage by uterine artery lagation. Timely intervention avoids hysterectomy and consumption coagulopathy and preserves reproductive potential.
- ✓ Retroperineal packing is a technique used by trauma surgeons to tamponade retroperitoneal hemorrhage related to pelvic fracture; it can also be useful to control retroperitoneal bleeding in obstetrical patients. Through a midline incision just above the symphysis pubis, the fascia is divided and the space of Retzius accessed, with care to avoid cystotomy. Two to three laparotomy sponges are placed sequentially in the retroperitoneal space, beginning at sacroiliac joint

and staying deep to the pelvic brim. The same procedure is then performed on the opposite side. The resulting tamponade generally leads to prompt cessation of blood loss. The packs are removed or exchanged 24 to 48 hours later, with care to avoid disruption of clot.

✓ Selective arterial embolization is an effective technique for the control of postpartum uterine hemorrhage and hemorrhage related to pelvic trauma. Case reports have also described successful percutaneous transcatheter identification and embolization of bleeding retroperitoneal vessels in postpartum women, generally after conventional suture and packing methods failure. We consider this procedure useful for the hemodynamically stable patient who has evidence of continued bleeding during recovery from delivery and in whom there is a high suspicion of retroperitoneal bleeding or has failed surgical intervention.

B. Gynecological Causes

Regarding gynecological causes, surgical procedures may lead to the injury of paracervical and paravaginal vessels, ovarian vessels, uterine artery or rarely external or internal iliac vessels with major blood loss.

Postoperative hemorrhage after gynecological surgery can produce a pelvic hematoma, losing a large amount of blood and sometimes requiring a blood transfusion. Massive hemorrhage is defined as acute blood with loss of more than 25 percent of total blood volume or bleeding that requires emergency intervention to save the patient's life. Careful inspection of all pedicles before abdominal closure is the best method to prevent postoperative hemorrhage.

The most common sites of major blood loss in the pelvis (cephalad to caulad) are: inferior vena cava, presacral veins, ovarian vessels, common and external iliac vessels, internal iliac vessels, parametrial and paracervical varicosities, bladder pillars and posterior bladder.

Diagnosis

The clinical manifestations of postoperative intraabdominal bleeding are tachycardia, hypotension, oliguria (urine output < 20 ml/hour), confusion and increasing abdominal pain.

Patients who undergo laparoscopic surgery may also present approximately 72 hours postoperatively with a drop in hemoglobin, and a large purplish discoloration or hematoma of a lower quadrant of the abdomen and/or ipsilateral flank. A CT scan will reveal a large hematoma within the abdominal wall, which may extend along muscle planes to the flank. The discoloration will resolve over 10 to 14 days, as the blood is absorbed. Presumably, a vessel in the anterior abdominal wall was injured, went into spasm, and then relaxed and bled at a later time until it became tamponaded. These patients do not have pain or discomfort.

Evaluation of a patient with suspected postoperative bleeding includes physical examination and assessment of vital signs and urine output. A laboratory evaluation should exclude a decreasing hematocrit or bleeding diathesis. Postoperative mobilization of fluids from the extravascular space can lead to a falling hematocrit level without ongoing bleeding.

The patient should be taken promptly to the examining room where the operative site is inspected (including the vaginal cuff if the patient has had an hysterectomy).

Management

Concerning to the management, if there is suspicion of postoperative hemorrhage, fluid resuscitation should be initiated and preparation made for possible surgical re-exploration. Large-bore intravenous access should be placed, isotonic fluids given (normal saline or Ringer lactate), a Foley catheter reinserted, and the patient is in fasting. Crystalloid fluids should be replaced in a 3:1 ratio of fluid:blood loss.

Bleeding from the vaginal cuff can usually be sutured in the examination room. Likewise, superficial bleeding from wound can be controlled by opening the wound and coagulating or suturing subcutaneous vessels.

Patients who are stable but anemic may be managed conservatively. Transfusion is given, if appropriate, and hemodynamic status, urine output, and hematocrit are monitored. Further evaluation and more aggressive management are indicated if there is suspicion of ongoing blood loss.

Surgical re-exploration – patients who are hemodynamically unstable or have an increasing abdominal girth should be surgically re-explored. An absolute indication for re-exploration is abdominal compartment syndrome. This can be caused by significant intraperitoneal or retroperitoneal bleeding resulting in raised intraabdominal pressure. The increased pressure can be transmitted to the pleural space causing a decrease in lung compliance and hypoxemia and a decrease in venous return. Decreased perfusion of the kidneys can lead to oliguria and renal failure. Computed tomography is useful to assess the location and amount of intra- or retroperitoneal blood collection.

Identification of bleeding source and control of bleeding proceeds as follows:

Pressure application— At the onset of intraoperative hemorrhage, apply pressure to the bleeding area. This helps to control acute bleeding and allows a moment to alert the rest of the operating room team that excessive bleeding is occurring. Immediate and ongoing communication with all members of the surgical team is essential to an efficient and effective response to intraoperative hemorrhage.

While securing hemostasis is critical, techniques must be used carefully in order to avoid tissue necrosis, organ injury, vascular thrombosis, fistula formation, or nerve dysfunction . Once the bleeding area is identified and tamponade applied, to identify the ureter and major vessels to avoid inadvertent injuries to these structures is necessary. Also, it is generally better to avoid leaving packs in place at venous bleeding sites due to risk of venous stasis and thrombosis. In some cases, it is better to apply continued pressure while waiting for a vascular or general surgeon or another gynecologist. Applying pressure to a large vessel (ie, aorta or common iliac) should be reserved for situations in which direct pressure to the bleeding site does not stop or significantly slow the bleeding. Attempts at repair of vessels without experience may worsen the injury, particularly in major retroperitoneal veins.

Identify and control localized bleeding — The most common sites of major blood loss in the pelvis (cephalad to caudad) are: inferior vena cava, presacral veins, ovarian vessels, common and external iliac vessels, internal iliac vessels, parametrial and paracervical varicosities, and the bladder pillars, and posterior bladder. To locate bleeding sites from one or more vessels, dissect the pelvic fascia surrounding the source of bleeding, identify vital structures (ie, vessels or viscera), and isolate and ligate the bleeding vessels.

Pelvic dissection — The vascular structures of the reproductive tract are contained within the tissues that surround the pelvic viscera, ie, the paravesical, pararectal, vesicovaginal, and rectovaginal spaces. Development of the appropriate space will often allow to control the bleeding, avoiding trauma to important pelvic structures.

Care should be taken during dissection, as the walls of the major veins are delicate and injury can cause brisk bleeding. Also, blunt dissection along the common iliac vein, inferior vena cava, pelvic sidewall or the presacral area can avulse small tributaries from larger veins with resultant high volume bleeding.

Surgeons who do not perform radical surgery may be less familiar with the paravesical and pararectal spaces. The paravesical space is bounded laterally by the external iliac vessels and medially by the obliterated hypogastric artery (medial umbilical ligament). Dissection of this space exposes the lateral portions of the bladder, vagina and rectum.

The pararectal space is bounded laterally by the internal iliac artery and medially by the ureter, and can be entered by incision of the pelvic peritoneum (and preferably the round ligament) lateral to the iliac vessels. Separation of the vessels and the ureter and dissection posteriorly and slightly medially exposes the proximal pelvic ureter, the internal iliac vessels and the rectum.

Retroperitoneal bleeding — If bleeding occurs, and the retroperitoneum is not open or the bleeding is behind the ovarian pedicle, apply direct pressure to the area of bleeding. If bleeding continues, a fast, bloodless approach to exposing this area is to open the peritoneum over the paracolic gutter and mobilize the colon medially. If the peritoneum is already open, then the bleeding source is identified and managed as outlined above.

Ligation — Isolate vessels prior to ligation. Placing sutures, clips, or coagulating multiple layer of tissue may injure surrounding structures.

a) *Small vessels* — Bleeding from small vessels may be controlled with coagulation, suture, or surgical clips.
b) *Large vessels* — The aorta, vena cava, and common and external iliac vessels perfuse the extremities. The extensive arterial collateral circulation in the peripheral pelvis allows ligation of most other large vessels in a nonirradiated pelvis. Coagulation is not adequate for larger vessels and clips may either fall off or cut into a vessel larger than the clip, thereby enlarging the defect. Placing multiple clips also makes it difficult to isolate and identify the bleeding site, so suturing the defect with a running 4-0 to 6-0 monofilament suture on a cardiovascular needle may be the best option.
c) *Large veins* — Venous bleeding can be difficult to control due to the relatively high volume of blood flowing through fragile, irregular veins. Gentle pressure with sponge sticks on either side of the venous injury is the most useful method to minimize blood loss.

In addition, the placement of hemoclips will often control venous bleeding. However, application of hemoclips to a "peg hole defect" (avulsion of the small veins that enter the anterior surface of the common iliac vein and the inferior vena cava) can reduce the caliber of the lumen and lead to coagulation and thrombosis.

Management of diffuse bleeding — There are several clinically important causes of diffuse bleeding, which must be addressed to assess the volume of bleeding and if there is flow at all operative surfaces.

Diffuse bleeding may indicate a possible bleeding diathesis, and should be treated medically. Alternatively, diffuse low volume bleeding which is concentrated in several small areas (eg, sites of prior dissection of adhesions) is likely from small venous sources and may be amenable to the use of topical hemostatic agents. When brisk diffuse bleeding arises suddenly in the presacral area, laceration of the presacral vessels should be suspected and immediately addressed.

A. *Topical hemostatic agents* — Small areas of low volume bleeding can be treated with topical hemostatic agents. Investigation of these agents has focused on vascular, cardiac, and hepatic surgery. There are few high quality data regarding treatment efficacy or use in gynecologic surgery. Thus, choices are made based on surgeon preference, availability, and cost-effectiveness.

- Gelatin — Gelatin (eg, Gelfoam®) is available in sponge or powder form . The sponge can be cut into any shape to facilitate application. Gelatin sponges are rigid when dry, but are pliable when moist and can be passed through laparoscopic ports. Pressure is applied for several minutes after application and the sponge is left in place. Gelatin is completely absorbed after four to six weeks with little tissue reaction or scarring. Disadvantages of gelatin include: increased incidence of infection, granuloma, and fibrosis formation as well as potential disruption of the clot if the sponge is removed. There is no data regarding the use of topical gelatin for hemostasis in gynecologic surgery. Although it is common practice to apply topical thrombin to gelatin matrix, in attempt to increase hemostasis, there is no consistent data to support this.
- Oxidized regenerated cellulose (ORC) — ORC (eg, Surgicel®) is supplied as a mesh and can be applied dry directly to bleeding areas. ORC is pliable, and can be rolled and passed easily through laparoscopic trocars. It requires a blood-free field to be effective. ORC takes 14 days to be fully absorbed . ORC also has bactericidal activity against a wide range of gram-positive and negative organisms. However, excessive use of ORC may

facilitate infection or adhesion formations. Successful use of ORC to control bleeding from small uterine perforations and tubal hemorrhage has been reported in small case series.

- ❖ Microfibrillar collagen (MC) — MC (eg, Avitene®) is an absorbable acid salt obtained from bovine collagen. MC is applied in powder form directly to the bleeding site using a dry, smooth forceps. MC is fully absorbed within three months. Although MC has low antigenicity, it may induce local edema. There is one case report of a systemic allergic reaction during a laparoscopic cholecystectomy associated with MC. Case reports of Holub Z use to show successful results in bleeding from uterine perforation and after hysterectomy; adverse effects noted include severe allergic reaction and granuloma formation.
- ❖ Topical thrombin (TT) — Bovine or human thrombin is used. Bovine thrombin is associated with anaphylaxis and the development of antibodies which can cross react with human factor V or human thrombin, leading to coagulopathy. In addition, there is a risk of infection transmission with human pooled plasma-derived thrombin. TT (eg, Thrombogen ®) can be applied via direct spray with a needle and syringe or in conjunction with a gelatin sponge in the surgical field. The use of thrombin has not been widely studied in gynecologic surgery.
- ❖ Fibrin sealant — Fibrin sealants (eg, Tisseel®) have two components that must be mixed prior to the application, one with thrombin and calcium chloride and other with concentrated fibrinogen, factor XIII, fibronectin, and fibrinolysis inhibitor. The mixture can then be directly sprayed onto bleeding sites. Fibrin sealants are used for hemostasis or as a tissue adhesive. This topic is discussed in more detail separately. There is one case report of transmission of parvovirus after use of a fibrin sealant for hemostasis during a hysterectomy.
- ❖ An autologous fibrin sealant (available in Europe, but not in the United States) showed a significantly higher rate of hemostasis (at 5 minutes after application) compared to ORC in a randomized trial on 69 patients undergoing obstetric, gynecologic, general, vascular, and cardiothoracic surgery.

B. *Presacral bleeding* — Laceration of the presacral plexus of veins and/or the middle sacral artery can lead to life-threatening hemorrhage. Pressing a sterile steel thumbtack directly into the bone at the bleeding site has been reported to be effective in observational studies ; the tack is not removed, and will show up on subsequent x-rays. Topical hemostatic agents, coagulation, clips, sutures, or bone may also control the bleeding . Another measure that has been reported is to excise and coagulate a piece of the rectus muscle and place it over the site of bleeding . As a last resort, an umbrella or parachute pack can be placed until the patient is stabilized .

Strategies for Persistent Bleeding

Internal iliac artery ligation — After initial failure attempts to achive hemostasis, the next step is to decrease pelvic blood flow. Bilateral internal iliac (hypogastric) artery ligation (IAL) lowers the pulse pressure of the pelvic vasculature by 85 percent and the rate of blood flow by 50 percent; low pressure systems are more amenable to clot formation.

IAL may help to avoid emergency hysterectomy. In a retrospective case series of patients with severe obstetric hemorrhage,published by Clark SL et al., 8 of 19 patients who underwent IAL did not undergo a subsequent hysterectomy. However, IAL precludes subsequent embolization. Therefore, it should be reserved for patients who are unlikely to be candidates for arterial embolization. The technique for IAL is performed bilaterally as follows:

1) Open the anterior leaf of the broad ligament (with a Metzenbaum scissors or electrosurgery) and lyse the areolar tissue of the retroperitoneum.
2) The external iliac artery is readily identified at the medial margin of the psoas muscle, and is followed to the common iliac artery bifurcation. The internal iliac artery is about 4 cm in length before it divides into anterior and posterior branches.
3) Ideally, the dissection should be carried caudally to the anterior and posterior trunks of the internal iliac artery so that the anterior trunk can be selectively ligated. In practice, this is so difficult that the entire internal iliac artery usually is ligated at its origin.
4) Dissect away the nodal tissue overlying the internal iliac artery by spreading the tissue with a right angle or tonsil clamp or the tips of Metzenbaum scissors. Continue the dissection anterior and lateral to the internal iliac artery. Proceed in the same plane around the circumference of the artery to separate it from the internal iliac vein, which is slightly medial and posterior to the artery. Pass a number 1

silk or nonabsorbable synthetic suture (eg, polypropylene) around the artery from lateral to medial and tie securely.

There are two important technical errors that are easy to commit, both of which may be detrimental:

- It is possible to mistakenly ligate the external iliac instead of the internal iliac artery. This usually leads to loss of the ipsilateral lower limb if not promptly corrected. Therefore, the lower limb (dorsalis pedis, or posterior tibial pulse) should be assessed for the presence of a pulse immediately after vessel ligation.
- The large, dilated, fragile internal iliac vein lies just behind and slightly medial to the artery and is often not visualized during isolation of the artery. Laceration of this vein can lead to rapid exsanguination. The external iliac artery lies lateral to the internal iliac artery and care should also be taken to avoid it.

A review of pregnancy outcome after internal iliac artery ligation for postpartum hemorrhage described 49 pregnancies with no evidence of any increase in adverse events.

Uterine artery ligation — Mass ligation of the uterine artery may be performed. The arteries are identified by palpation. To ligate the left uterine artery, the uterus is elevated upwards and to the right. A large blunt needle with #0 or #1 absorbable suture is passed into and through the myometrium about 2 cm medial to and below the uterine vessels. The needle is brought out through the avascular area in the broad ligament, cephalad and lateral to left uterine vessels, and the suture is tied. The procedure is repeated on the contralateral side.

Hysterectomy or oophorectomy — If bleeding continues despite conservative measures, removal of the adnexae or uterus may be necessary despite the initial surgical plan. For example, in women undergoing myomectomy or ovarian cystectomy who develop intractable bleeding, the possibility of emergency measures in case of hemorrhage is part of the preoperative consent process.

Prolonged pelvic packing — If other measures do not control bleeding, a pressure pack may be left in the pelvis for 48 to 72 hours. The patient is monitored closely and appropriate fluid resuscitation and blood transfusion administered in an intensive care setting. Packs may be removed via the vaginal cuff or by re-opening the laparotomy. Our approach to pelvic packing in a patient who had a hysterectomy is as follows:

- Fill a large sterile drawstring-closure plastic bag with three rolls of gauze tied end-to-end; leave the tail of the gauze protruding through the bag's opening and tighten the drawstrings. Place the pack is in the pelvis, avoiding bowel or ovary entrapment. Pull the drawstrings and gauze tail through the vaginal cuff. A 1000 mL intravenous fluid bag is attached to the pack with surgical tubing and hung off the end of the bed for traction. Place a Jackson-Pratt drain in the pelvis to monitor for continued bleeding and an indwelling urinary catheter to avoid outflow obstruction and monitor urine output.
- After 48 to 72 hours, if vaginal and Jackson-Pratt drainage have decreased, remove the gauze through the vagina, slowly over four hours. The bag can then be removed through the vagina and the vaginal cuff left open.

Other measures — The use of medical anti-shock trousers or garments is controversial. While a few case reports and a small case series report successful use in gynecologic and obstetric hemorrhage, an animal study of intraabdominal hemorrhage found that these devices did not slow bleeding.

Embolization — Embolization halts pelvic bleeding by occluding pelvic arteries. This is an option for patients in whom volume status can be maintained until the procedure can be completed (approximately two hours). As discussed above, ligation of the internal iliac artery will preclude subsequent embolization.

Preoperative embolization has been used for procedures where the risk of hemorrhage is felt to be high.

Percutaneous transcatheter embolization procedures are performed under fluoroscopic guidance in the radiology suite with intravenous conscious sedation, analgesics, and antibiotic prophylaxis. Gelfoam, coils, and glue are preferred for embolization of large arteries and tiny particles or microspheres are preferred for small arteries.

Postpartum hemorrhage in hemodynamically stable patients can be managed with percutaneous transcatheter embolization. Consultation with an interventional radiologist should be obtained early to facilitate decision making. The physician needs to consider that if embolization is unsuccessful, uterine artery ligation can be attempted subsequently. In contrast, embolization may be extremely difficult, or even impossible, after an unsuccessful uterine artery ligation.

3) Endografts — Patients with postoperative bleeding due to injury to the vena cava or common or external iliac veins may be candidates for placement of stented grafts by an endovascular specialist.

C. Other Causes

Other causes of pelvic hematoma include trauma, anticoagulation, ruptured ectopic pregnancy, and rupture of an aneurysm in the abdominopelvic vasculature.These cases need to be treated by solving the etiology which has caused the bleeding.

References

Achneck HE, Sileshi B, Jamiolkowski RM, Albala DM, Shapiro ML, Lawson JH. A comprehensive review of topical hemostatic agents: efficacy and recommendations for use. *Ann. Surg.* 2010;251(2):217.

Benrubi G, Neuman C, Nuss RC, Thompson RJ. Vulvar and vaginal hematomas: a retrospective study of conservative versus operative management. *South Med. J.* 1987; 80:991.

Burchell RC. Physiology of internal iliac artery ligation. *J. Obstet. Gynaecol. Br. Commonw.* 1968; 75:642.

Burchell RC. Physiology of internal iliac artery ligation. *J. Obstet. Gynaecol. Br. Commonw.* 1968;75(6):642.

Clark SL, Phelan JP, Yeh SY, Bruce SR, Paul RH. Hypogastric artery ligation for obstetric hemorrhage. *Obstet. Gynecol.* 1985;66(3):353.

Duenas-Garcia OF, Goldberg JM. Topical hemostatic agents in gynecologic surgery. *Obstet. Gynecol. Surv.* 2008;63(6):389.

Evans S, McShane P. The efficacy of internal iliac artery ligation in obstetric hemorrhage. *Surg. Gynecol. Obstet.* 1985;160(3):250.

Fadi M , Sreedhar G. Obstetric emergencies. *Semin. Perinatol.* 2009; 33:97-103.

Gemer O, Shenhav S, Segal S, Harari D, Segal O, Zohav E. Sonographically diagnosed pelvic hematomas and postcesarean febrile morbility. *International Journal of Gynecology and Obstetrics* 1999;65:7-9.

Gostout BS, Cliby WA, Podratz KC. Prevention and management of acute intraoperative bleeding. *Clin. Obstet. Gynecol.* 2002;45(2):481.

Hansch E, Chitkara U, McAlpine J. Pelvic arterial embolization for control of obstetric hemorrhage: a five-year experience. *Am. J. Obstet. Gynecol* 1999; 180:145.

Hebisch G, Huch A. Vaginal uterine artery ligation avoids high blood loss and puerperal hysterectomy in postpartum hemorrhage. *Obstet Gynecol.* 2002;100(3):574-8.

Holub Z, Jabor A. Laparoscopic management of bleeding after laparoscopic or vaginal hysterectomy. *JSLS.* 2004;8(3):235.

Hong YM, Loughlin KR. The use of hemostatic agents and sealants in urology. *J. Urol.* 2006;176(6 Pt 1):2367.

Howard RJ, Straughn JM Jr, Huh WK, Rouse DJ. Pelvic umbrella pack for refractory obstetric hemorrhage secondary to posterior uterine rupture. *Obstet. Gynecol.* 2002;100(5 Pt 2):1061.

Morita Y, Nishii O, Kido M, Tsutsumi O. Parvovirus infection after laparoscopic hysterectomy using fibrin glue hemostasis. *Obstet. Gynecol.* 2000;95(6 Pt 2):1026.

Nizard J, Barrinque L, Frydman R, Fernandez H. Fertility and pregnancy outcomes following hypogastric artery ligation for severe post-partum haemorrhage. *Hum. Reprod.* 2003;18(4):844.

Sheikh GN. Perinatal genital hematomas. *Obstet. Gynecol.* 1971; 38:571.

Smith WR, Moore EE, Osborn P. Retroperitoneal packing as a resuscitation technique for hemodynamically unstable patientswith pelvic fractures: report of two representative cases and a description of technique. K *Trauma* 2005; 59:1510.

Yamashita Y, Torashima M, Harada M, Yamamoto H, Takahashi M. Postpartum Extraperitoneal Pelvic Hematoma: Imaging. *AJR* 1993; 161:805-808.

Zahn CM, Hankins GD, Yeomans ER, Vulvovaginal hematomas complicating delivery. Rationale for drainage of the hematoma cavity. *J. Reprod. Med.* 1996; 41: 569.

In: Hematomas: Types, Treatments … ISBN: 978-1-61942-385-5
Editors: M.F.G.Salazar…pp. 143-169

Chapter V

"Intracraneal Hematomas in Pediatric Patient"

***Roberto Velasco Zúñiga*[1], *Helvia Benito Pastor*[1] *and Maria Elena Vilacastín Ruiz*[2]**
[1]Pediatrics Department, Río Hortega Teaching Hospital, Valladolid, Spain
[2]Radiology Department, Río Hortega Teaching Hospital, Valladolid, Spain

1. Introduction

An intracranial hematoma is a collection of blood in the head. The etiology is often traumatic, but can also occur in non-traumatic conditions as in the case of coagulopathy, metabolic diseases, vascular anomalies, or as a result of rupture of previously asymptomatic intracranial cysts. Depending the location, intracranial hematomas present with different symptoms and require different management, so it is important to recognize the symptoms to reach a diagnosis and to treatment as soon as possible. So, depending the location of hematomas we could classify them as:

- Epidural: located between the dura and the bone. Generally caused by head trauma.
- Subdural: located between the dura and the arachnoid membranes. Also caused by trauma more oftenly.

- Subarachnoid: located between the arachnoid membranes and the brain. Trauma is also the most common cause of subarachnoid hemorrhage (SAH), but spontaneous is not infrequent. The main cause is rupture of an aneurysm or a cerebral arteriovenous malformation (AVM).
- Intracerebral: located in the brain parenchyma. Caused more frequently by ruptured AVM. Also frequent to found it in premature infants.
- Inraventricular: located inside the cerebral ventricules. Most frequently associated to hypoxic-ischemic encephalopathy.

Epidural Hematoma

Common locations are frontal, parietooccipital and more often, posterior fossa, unlike adult population, in which temporal is the most common location. The source of bleeding in posterior fossa is venous.

Symptoms are caused by mass effect on the brain, and the increased intracranial pressure.

Classic presentation is an altered mental status, decreased level of conciousness, seizures, vomiting, etc. after a head injury, with or without a "lucid interval".

The first approach to the patient must include physical examination of the head, looking for external injuries or wounds, and neurologic examination (Glasgow scale score (GCS), papillary findings, craneal nerves and cerebelar exploration).

The gold standard of diagnostic imaging is the head CT. If there is a hematoma, usually appears as a biconvex or lenticular hyperdense mass between brain and bone.

Treatment is more often surgical. If the hematoma is larger of 10 mm of thickness, or there are any physical finding as papillary abnormalities, hemiparesis, GCS < 8 or sudden fall of 2 or more points related to admission, seizures or cerebelar signs; an emergent craniotomy should be done.

Nonsurgical treatment could be made in asymptomatic patients with small hematomas, always under close vigilance.

When early evacuation of hematoma is made, outcomes are usually favourable. Mortality is about 2-6% cases.

Subdural Hematoma

Usually caused by trauma, in children < 2 years of age abusive head injury should be considered. Any location is possible, but hematomas associated with abusive head injury are more often located in the interhemispheric space and the posterior fossa.

Clinical features are similar to epidural hematomas. In patients under 2 years of age, symptoms could be unspecific, as irritability, lethargy, vomiting, full or protuberant anterior fontanelle, increased head circumference, etc.

Physical examination must be very conscientious looking for findings suggestive of children abuse, like hematomas in other body parts, burn lesions, retinal hemorrages, genital injuries, etc.

As in epidural hematomas, gold standard for diagnosis is head CT.

There is no clear criteria for surgical treatment. Decision of sending patient under surgery is taken based in clinical an imaging features, considering every patient individually.

Outcome is mainly based on neurologic state of patient at admission.

2. Epidural Hemorrhage

2.1. Introduction

The dura coats the inside of the skull and also forms the periosteum. From it come away strong walls into the skull. The falx is in the sagittal plane separating the two cerebral hemispheres. Ii inserts rostrally in the crista galli apophysis and in the frontal crest and, following the course of the superior sagittal sinus, reached the internal occipital protuberance caudally, where it merges with the tentorium, which extends to both sides. The falx divides the top of the cranial cavity so that each hemisphere is kept in their own space. The tentorium covers the cerebellum housed in the posterior cranial fossa. It is inserted along the groove of the transverse occipital sinus, and in the top edge of the left petrous temporal and leaves orally an opening for the passage of the brainstem. The falx of the cerebellum projects to the posterior cranial fossa from the underside of the tentorium and the occipital crest. The dural sinuses are included between two layers of dura [1].

When a head injury happens, the bone may be depressed into the head, separating dura from the bone, thereby creating a space in which blood collects. Because of the strong walls that attach the dura to the bone, it is unlikely that an epidural hematoma cross the cranial sutures.

In infants and young children, the source of bleeding is usually venous. By coming off the dura from the bone is injured a venous sinus or some bridging vein.

In older children and adolescents the origin is similar to that of adults, usually the lesion in some branch of the middle meningeal artery by a bone fragment.

2.2. Etiology

An epidural hematoma is seen in 1-3% of admissions from traumatic brain closed injury (TBI). They are more common in males, with a ratio of 2-2,5:1 [2].

The etiology is usually age-dependent:

- In newborns epidural hematomas are rare and the few that occur are usually associated with instrumental delivery.
- In infants and children are frequent hematomas caused by falls. In short fall (<1 m) less than 1% of patients have an epidural hematoma. However, 50% of children who fell from a fifth or sixth floor died, 78% of them due to head injury [3].
- In adolescents, the vast majority are caused by motor vehicle collision [2].

2.3. Pathophysiology

Location of the hematoma is different in children than in adults. In adults, hematomas are quite common in the temporal region. However, the temporal artery in the child is not so close to the bone, so do not get hurt so easily.

As we have said, falls are the leading cause of epidural hematoma in infancy, so a vast majority of injuries occur on the occipital region, with the greater incidence of fractures and, secondarily, also incidence of hematomas, although only 3% of children with occipital fracture developed epidural hematoma in this region[4]. At this location, the bleeding is usually venous, so the accumulation of blood will be slower, resulting in a period of time the child is asymptomatic, which is known as the *lucid interval*, followed by a rapid neurological deterioration.

Other typical locations of epidural hematomas in children are the frontal and parietooccipital fossas.

When there is an epidural hematoma, it increases intracranial pressure. In children, once the cranial sutures are closed, cranial volume becomes constant. From this moment, intracranial pressure depends on the volume of intracranial structures, that is the brain (80% of intracranial volume), blood (10%) and cerebrospinal fluid (10%).

By increasing the volume of the hematoma, it shifts first fluids, such as cerebrospinal fluid and blood, making cerebral perfusion difficult, and if it continues increasing, finally shifts the brain parenchyma and may cause herniation of it through the foramen magnum.

In children who still have open fontanel, increasing intracranial pressure is better tolerated. This may cause the amount of accumulated blood without causing neurologic symptoms is higher, it can produce hypovolemia clinic even before neurological symptoms [2].

Some authors suggest intracranial pressure limits for the start of treatment according to the age of child [5]:

- 15 mmHg in less than one year
- 18 mmHg in children between 1 and 8 years
- 20 mmHg over 8 years.

2.4. Symptomatology

An epidural hematoma must be suspected in any patient with an altered state of consciousness following a traumatic brain injury (TBI). Some data from medical records can increase our level of suspicion, as a high-impact head injury, the presence of a lucid interval or a preexisting coagulopathy.

Symptoms that should make us suspect an epidural hematoma is an altered level of consciousness, headache, repeated vomiting or the presence of seizures. In large hematomas the patient may present in a coma. We must watch for signs of lateralizing, as anisocoria, hemiparesis or hemiplegia, suggesting a progression to brain herniation. The pupil size is directly proportional to the hematoma in more than 90% of cases [2]. Cushing triad (bradycardia, hypertension and bradypnea) presentation is usually late and often indicates an imminent irreversible deterioration.

In infants with open fontanel, as already mentioned, neurological symptoms may be delayed, and sometimes we see symptoms associated with hypovolemia, such as paleness, irritability, tachycardia, or sweating. We can find a large cephalohematoma in the region of the trauma. In these patients the presence of Cushing triad is always associated with a poor prognosis.

In neonates it is not surprising that first symptoms are hypotonia or seizures.

Between 37-67% of patients may experience a lucid interval. The child shows an impaired level of consciousness immediately after injury, followed by a recovery of normal level of consciousness, and once the cumulative amount of blood is enough to compress the brain, the child shows rapid impairment.

In occipital trauma, being generally the source of bleeding venous, the clinic could be subacute. They tend to associate an initial loss of consciousness followed by headache and / or vomiting. Later, they can present dizziness, stiff neck or cerebellar signs such as ataxia, dysarthria, tremor, or pyramidal sygns. Neurological deterioration in these patients may be faster than in other hematomas due to the limited space of the posterior fossa, and the possible involvement of the brainstem, or possible hydrocephalus by compression of the fourth ventricle.

2.5. Management

2.5.1. Primary Survey

The initial management of head injuries is the same in all polytrauma patient.

In the primary survey and stabilization of trauma patients must be followed in an order that is outlined by the letters ABCDE [6.]

A. Airway Stabilization and Cervical Immobilization:

- Head must be maintained in neutral position without traction.
- If the airway is open only administer 100% O_2.
- If the airway is closed shall be its opening with standard CPR procedures. The safest method for opening the airway in a child with possible cervical spine injury is the jaw thrust.

If you can not secure the airway, proceed to intubation, which is indicated in cases of ineffective breathing, severe bradycardia, Glasgow <8 or hemodynamic instability.

B. Breathing. Ventilation

All trauma patients must be stabilized with 100% O_2. If the patient is breathing spontaneously proceed to gastric decompression with nasopharyngeal tube and administer O_2 with nasal cannula or mask.

If the patient is in apnea will proceed to bag-mask ventilation or intubation if necessary.

C. Circulation: Control of Shock and Hemorrhage

In this phase is crucial a clinical evaluation based on of peripheral perfusion, quality and intensity of the pulse and heart rate. First, we must control external bleeding by compression, and think about the internal bleeding.

If there is shock get 1 or 2 peripheral venous access. If not achieved at the second attempt will proceed to the intraosseous access. Once channeled be administered isotonic crystalloid (Ringer lactate or saline serum) 20cc/Kg in 10-15 minutes. If no improvement is seen there will be a second infusion at 10-20 cc / kg, and if it does not respond should continue with isotonic colloid (5% Serum albumin + Saline serum) 10-20 cc / kg and consider transfusion.

D. Disability. Neurological Assessment

Having stabilized the patient's cardiorespiratory function will be a brief neurological evaluation. It will check the level of consciousness by the Glasgow Coma Scale (GCS) age-appropriate (Table 1), will be assessed pupillary abnormalities and brain stem reflexes. If the situation is not extremely urgent, it will also explore the cranial nerves, motor function and cerebellar exploration [5].

If after initial assessment neurological injury or increased intracranial ICP are suspected, measures to reduce the risk of secondary brain injury has been taken:

- Administer O_2 needed to maintain peripheral O_2 saturation> 95%
- Maintain cervical immobilization until the imaging studies demonstrate the absence of bone injury. If the patient is unconscious,

keep restraint regardless of the outcome of imaging tests until you wake up and check that it is asymptomatic.

- If the patient has needed intubation, avoid excessive hyperventilation, trying to keep $PaCO_2$ all the time between 35 and 40 mmHg, as otherwise hypocarbia could cause decreased cerebral blood flow that could cause cerebral ischemia.
- Hypotension must be adequately treated, to maintain adequate cerebral perfusion. We recommend a cerebral perfusion pressure (mean arterial pressure - ICP) above 60 mmHg [7]. In a recent study, appropriate for age systolic blood pressure (AASBP) $<P_{75}$ was associated with a worse prognosis, although systolic pressure was greater than 90 mmHg [8].
- Fit an intracranial pressure sensor in all patients with Glasgow <8 [5].

Table 1. Glasgow Coma Scale and Glasgow Coma Scale modified for infants

Glasgow scale		Glasgow scale modified for infants	
Activity	Better response	Activity	Better response
Eye opening		*Eye opening*	
Spontaneously	4	Spontaneously	4
To voice	3	To voice	3
To pain	2	To pain	2
No response	1	No response	1
Verbal		*Verbal*	
Oriented	5	Babbling, smile, cry	5
Confused	4	Continous crying	4
Inappropriate words	3	Inappropiate crying	3
Incomprehensible sounds	2	Grunts	2
No verbal response	1	No verbal response	1
Motor		*Motor*	
Obbey commands	6	Spontaneous movements	6
Localizes pain	5	Localizes pain	5
Flexion/withdrawal to pain	4	Flexion/withdrawal to pain	4
Abnormal flexion to pain (decorticate response)	3	Abnormal flexion to pain (decorticate response)	3
Extension to pain (decerebrate response)	2	Extension to pain (decerebrate response)	2
No movements	1	No movements	1

E. Exposure

All trauma patients should be stripped completely for a full recognition that allows the discovery of lesions that have slipped past.

2.5.2. Laboratory And Image Tests:

Blood test should be done to rule out anemia due to bleeding or coagulopathy. This will involve a complete blood count (CBC) with platelet count and a coagulation study. In these patients should always take blood for crossing about the possibility of needing a blood transfusion.

It is not recommended to perform a lumbar puncture in these patients, given the possibility of an high intracranial pressure, which increases the risk of herniation because of removing cerebrospinal fluid.

The cornerstone of diagnosis in these patients are imaging tests:

- **Radiography**: skull radiography should be performed in all children under 2 years of age whom fell from more than ½ metre high, collision with vehicle speed, impact on hard surface or trauma with a blunt or heavy object, or presence of an important cephalohematoma. In case of skull fracture evident on the radiograph should undergo a cranial CT, as in children under 2 years old skull fractures associate with more frequency intracranial hematomas [7].
  In 1-3% of children with low impact TBI skull fracture is evident. Fractures are usually linear, and less than 1% associated intracranial hematoma [3].
- **Transfontanelar ultrasound**: In infants the fontanelles remain open, so it is possible doing an ultrasound instead of CT, thereby limiting radiation. However, this technique has limited sensitivity in case of epidural or subdural hematomas located in craneal convexities [9].
- **Transcranial Doppler**: provides information on cerebral blood flow. Is useful in patients with severe head injuries. In these patients, diastolic velocity in the middle cerebral artery of less than 25 $cm \cdot s^{-1}$ is associated with poor neurologic outcome [10].
- **Head CT**: is the main diagnostic method, given its rapid implementation. Epidural hematomas are often seen as a biconvex or lentiform mass that separates the brain from the skull, always respecting the suture lines. In most cases appear as a hyperdense mass (Figure 1), although up to a third part of them may be seen as hypo- and hyperdense areas interspersed. Hypodense areas usually are unclotted blood, indicating active bleeding.
  CT can delimit the location of the hematoma, helping for surgical approach. In addition, in CT indirect signs of increased intracranial pressure can be observed, as a shift from the midline, collapse of the lateral ventricle ipsilateral to the lesion, or collapse of the basal

cisterns. It may also be seen lost of differentiation between white matter and gray matter, suggestive of cerebral edema, or signs of herniation.

- **MRI scan:** is considered the most sensitive method for detection of intracranial hematomas [11], but is rarely used in the acute phase because it is slower than the CT. Its use is restricted to monitoring patients, or those cases with high clinical suspicion of hematoma and normal CT (Figure 2).
- **Angiography:** rarely used except in cases of suspected vascular malformation.

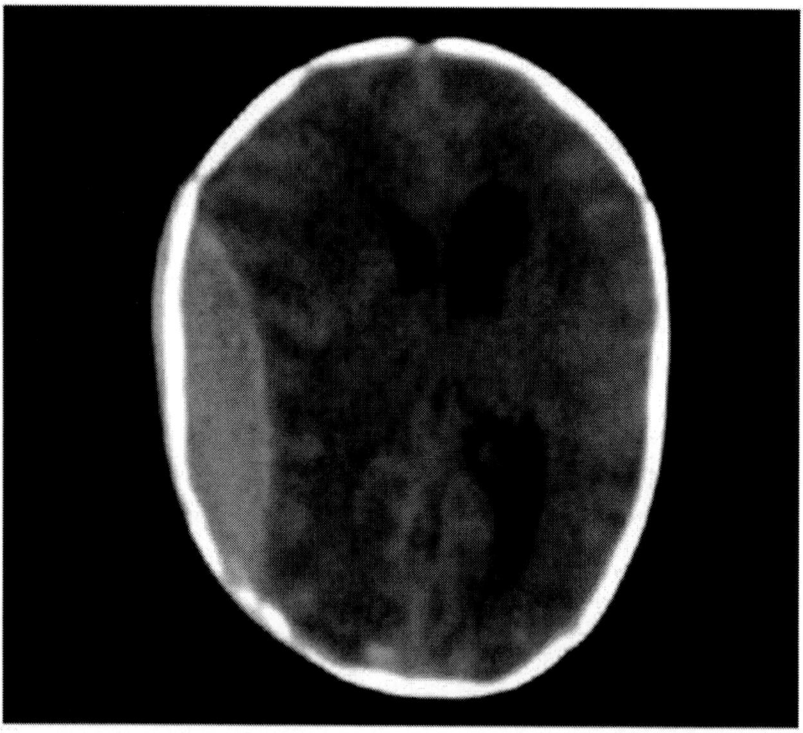

Figure 1. CT scan without contrast. Collection intracranial, extra-axial biconvex, hyperdense, consistent with acute epidural hematoma. Produce discrete contralateral shift of midline and compression of the occipital horn of right lateral ventricle.

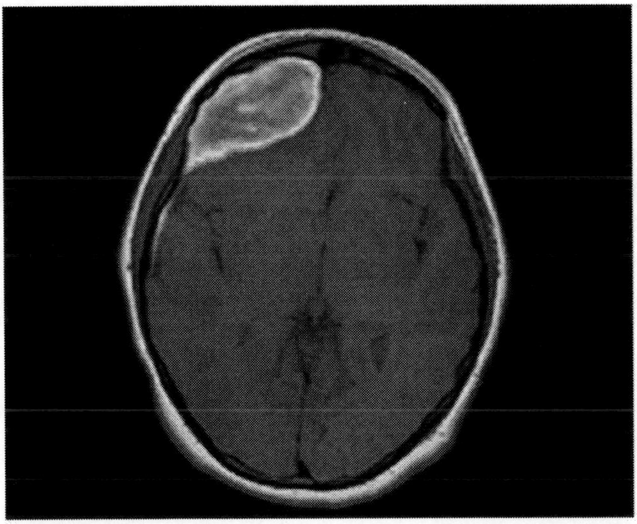

Figure 2. MRI axial T1. Biconvex extra-axial collection compatible with right frontal epidural hematoma. It is noted that conditions contralateral shift of the midline (subfalcine herniation).

2.5.3. Hematoma Treatment

In most cases the treatment is surgical. Only in very select cases you can choose nonoperative management. They must meet ALL of the following conditions:

- Thick of hematoma less than <10 mm
- Location different than the temporal region
- Volume of less than 30 cc
- Shift of the midline <5 mm
- GCS > 8
- No focal signs

These criteria are even stricter in the posterior fossa hematomas because the less space in this area, and the risk of complication is greater [4].

Nonoperative management includes admission and close observation. A CT scan must be done within 24 hours. If at any time the patient develops signs of local mass effect, herniation signs (lethargy, pupillary changes, hemiparesis, etc.) emergency surgical drainage of the hematoma should be performed.

Patients with small hematomas that remain asymptomatic in 24-48 hours of admission can be discharged.

If the patient does not meet all the criteria, surgical drainage of the hematoma should be performed. The goals of surgery are removal of the clot, proper hemostasis of bleeding and prevent reaccumulation of blood. Decompressive craniectomy has shown better results than burr holes. Pediatric patients show a better prognosis after decompressive surgery than adults [12,13].

2.6. Follow-Up and Outcome

A head CT should be performed in a month after injury. If there are not anomalies and the patient is asymptomatic, follow-up could be resumed at this point. If not, individualized following will be established for each patient.

Patients with neurological deficits should be referred to occupational therapy as early as possible [14].

The most important factor in neurological outcome of epidural hematomas in children is the time between the onset of impaired conciousness and the evacuation of hematoma [14].

The signs found on physical examination that are associated more strongly with brain injuries are: suspected open fracture, signs of fracture of the skull base, large hematoma, low score on the Glasgow Coma Scale or damage it during the stay in the ED.

Patients with high GCS at presentation, without pupillary changes and absence of associated cerebral injuries have better outcome.

3. Subdural Hemorrhage

3.1. Introduction

The arachnoid membrane is an avascular structure, web-shaped, attached to the inside of the dura[A]. Between the dura and the arachnoid, is a layer of flat cells formed by fibroblasts with intercellular junctions, known as subdural space. This is not a virtual space, but a compartment formed by a tissue between the two meninges. When the blood is collected in that area, do not fill a space but occupies a tissue in which breaks the intercellular joints [15]. When blood collects in this space, makes a subdural hematoma.

3.2. Etiology

The etiology of these conditions changes with age:

- In **neonates** is rare to see these pathology, and are usually associated with delivery labour. However, it is more common to find subarachnoid hematomas [16].
- **Infants**: incidence in children under 1 year is 20-25 cases per 100,000 children / year, and 12 cases per 100,000 children / year in children under 2 years old [17]. Most cases are due to inflicted trauma. The incidence of inflicted brain injury in USA is 1 / 3367 children / year [18]. It is estimated that half of the TCE that cause death or irreversible sequelae in infants are secondary to intentional harm.
- In **older children**, the main cause, as in epidural hematomas, are high-energy trauma, mainly collisions with motor vehicles.

In most cases, subdural hematomas result from bleeding caused by tearing one of the bridging veins as a result of rotational and deceleration forces produced in a head injury. Sometimes the source of bleeding is cerebral cortex as a result of direct trauma.

In infants with inflicted injury by direct trauma or shaken vigorously, a separation may occur between the gray and white matter, and rupture of bridging veins by the sudden movement of the brain inside the skull.

Hematomas may also be secondary to infectious processes that may injure the vessels (i.e. meningitis), conditions that predispose to bleeding (coagulopathy), or processes increasing extra-axial space, such as glutaric aciduria type 1.

Sometimes a sudden drop in intracranial pressure by draining the CSF may cause a decrease in the brain, which pulls the dura, being able to rip some bridging vein and cause a subdural hematoma. This condition is usually iatrogenic, sometimes secondary to ventricle-peritoneal shunt in a patient with hydrocephaly [19], or performing a lumbar puncture in a patient with intracranial hypertension.

It is unusual that hematoma to be pure blood. In most cases it is blood mixed with fluid [4].

As with epidural hematoma, location is the most diverse. Hematomas associated to injuries often locate in the convexities of the frontal, parietal and temporal lobes. In children under 2 years of accidental origin, 75% are bilateral or have contralateral fluid collections [4]. The location in the posterior fossa is rare, in contrast to the epidural hematomas [20].

A subdural hematoma located in the interhemispheric space, or multiple hematomas suggest inflicted trauma [4].

3.3. Pathophysiology

Pathophysiology of subdural hematomas is similar than epidural hematoma (see *epidural hematoma pathophysiology*).

The source of bleeding and severity of brain injury are related to the type of injury:

- **Severe head injury**: after a severe head injury, such as a motor vehicle collision the bleeding comes from tearing of the bridging veins, but also from an extensive damage to the cerebral cortex. The radiographic subdural hematoma image may be small, but is accompanied by signs of diffuse brain injury. In these cases, the morbidity and mortality are much higher than would correspond to larger hematomas caused by less impact mechanisms. Generally, subdural hematomas caused by high-energy trauma have a worse prognosis than epidurals because of the associated brain damage.
- **Inflicted head injury (shaken baby syndrome):** infants have special characteristics that make them more susceptible to this type of injury. On the one hand, a relatively larger head with more extra-axial space and a higher content in water of the brain, along with hypotonia of the neck muscles, make children of this age much more susceptible to injury from acceleration -deceleration mechanism. Moreover, in these patients medical care is often delayed, sothis patients usually have hypoxic-ischemic lesions associated.
- **Minor head injury**: in the low-energy trauma the source of bleeding is often the rupture of some bridging vein, with no associated cortical injury. In these cases, the hematoma can be larger, with less symptoms, since the blood accumulates slowly. Sometimes the source of bleeding is the rupture of some arteriovenous malformation, or an arachnoid cyst [21].

After the initial trauma a collagen synthesis is induced in the dura, and fibroblasts lining the inside of the membrane, forming a new thicker outer membrane. Following this, a thin inner membrane completely encapsulates the clot. This takes place within about two weeks.

Later, a chronic subdural hematoma can liquidify, or form a hygroma, and membranes may calcify. More than a half of chronic liquidified hematomas tend to increase in size, rather than solidify and remain stable. This is more common the larger the initial hematoma was.

Anytime the hematoma could increase its size secondary to a rebleeding or the osmotic entry of water into the hygroma due to its high protein content.

3.4. Symptomatology

As with epidural hematoma, a subdural hematoma must be suspected in any patient with altered neurological status after trauma (see *epidural hematoma symptomatology*)

Certain data from the clinical history may suggest the presence of a subdural hematoma in patients with unintentional injuries, such as a high-energy trauma (fall from more than 3 times the height of the patient or a motor vehicle crash), coagulopathy, cerebral atrophy or hydrocephalus, osteogenesis imperfecta, glutaric aciduria type 1, presence of an arachnoid cyst, etc.

Inflicted injury, should be suspected in cases of infants when the clinical history does not refer to a mechanism of injury that justifies the exploratory findings, when a is delay not justifiable in attendance, when strange parental attitudes or behavior are observed in infants (rejection of physical contact with parents or irritability and tranquility with the medical staff) [7]. The reason for consultation in patients with inflicted brain damage is often not a head injury, but presenting with clinical of apparent life-threatening event (ALTE), vomiting without diarrhea, seizures, or nonspecific neurological symptoms such as lethargy [18]. At other times the reason for consultation will be coma or cardiac arrest.

In physical exam of children under 2 years must always look for signs of physical abuse, including geometric injuries, in relatively protected areas or at different evolutionary stage, presence of other fractures and retinal hemorrhages [6].

In children with accidental head injury subdural hematoma may manifest as an altered mental status or focal neurological signs. Other findings may be a full fontanel or a sudden increase in head circumference.

Children with open fontanel can accumulate large amounts of blood prior to the presence of neurological symptoms. In these cases the neurological symptoms may be preceded by fever or signs of hypovolemia (paleness, tachycardia), or even of hemorrhagic shock.

Pupillary abnormalities and Cushing triad are late signs, and mean poor prognosis. Usually are followed by rapid neurological deterioration.

3.5. Treatment

3.5.1. Primary Survey

The initial management of head injuries is the same in all patients with multiple injuries (see *Epidural hematomas primary survey*).

3.5.2. Laboratory and Image Tests

Blood test should be done to rule out anemia due to bleeding or coagulopathy. This will involve a CBC with platelet count and a coagulation study. In these patients should always take blood for cross about the possibility of needing a blood transfusion.

It is not recommended to perform a lumbar puncture in these patients, given the possibility that the intracranial pressure is elevated, which increases the risk of herniation because of removing cerebrospinal fluid.

The cornerstone of diagnosis in these patients, as in the epidural hematomas, are image tests:

- **Radiography**: skull x-ray should be performed of all children under 2 years of age fell more than 1 meter of height, high-energy trauma or presence of important cephalohematoma. In case of skull fracture evident on the radiograph, patient should undergo a head CT, because in children under 2 years skull fractures are most commonly associated with intracranial hematomas.
  In addition, in suspected cases of physical abuse, complete skeleton X-ray will be done in search of skull or other bones fractures [22].
- **Transfontanelar ultrasound**: In infants the fontanelles remain open, so an ultrasound can be done instead of CT, thereby limiting radiation (figure 3). However, this technique has limited sensitivity in the case of epidural or subdural hematomas located in the craniofacial convexities [9].

- **Head CT**: is the main diagnostic method, given its rapid implementation. Subdural hematomas are often seen as a concave mass along the brain surface, not limited by the cranial sutures. Most of the hematomas caused by accidental trauma are often seen as a hyperdense mass (Figures 4 to 6). In those where attention is deferred, hypodense and hyperdense areas may be interspersed. In these cases, physical abuse should be suspected.
  If we find hemorrhages in several locations, or a hematoma that covers both hemispheres, we must almost unequivocally suspect that this is an child abuse situation[4].
  Depending on the degree of brain injury and size of the hematoma, uncal, transtentorial or subfalcina herniation may be associated, as well as other radiological signs of ischemia or hypoxia, such as loss of differentiation between gray and white matter. They may also be signs of concussion or subarachnoid hemorrhage [23].
- **MRI:** is considered the most sensitive method for detection of intracranial hematomas [11], but is rarely used in the acute phase because it is slower than the CT. Its use is restricted to follow-up of patients, or those cases with high clinical suspicion of hematoma and normal CT.

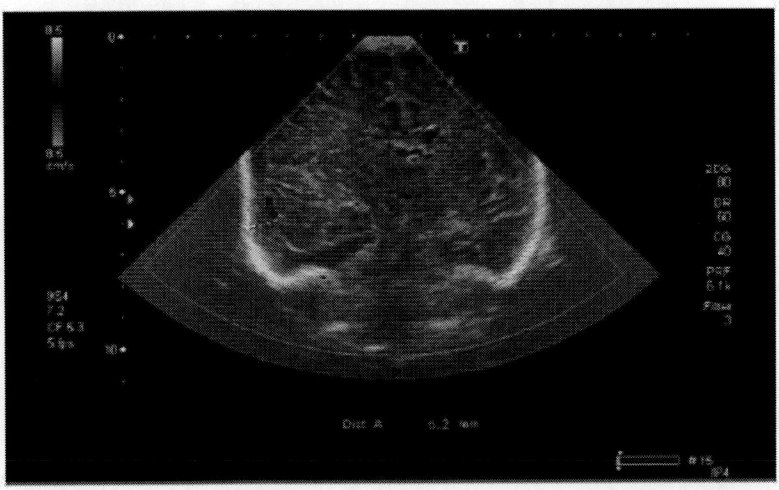

Figure 3. Transfontanelar ultrasound, coronal image. Extraaxial hypoechoic collection that spans the parietal region and right tentorium. Corresponds to a subacute subdural hematoma. It causes contralateral shift of the midline and partial collapse of the frontal horn of right lateral ventricle.

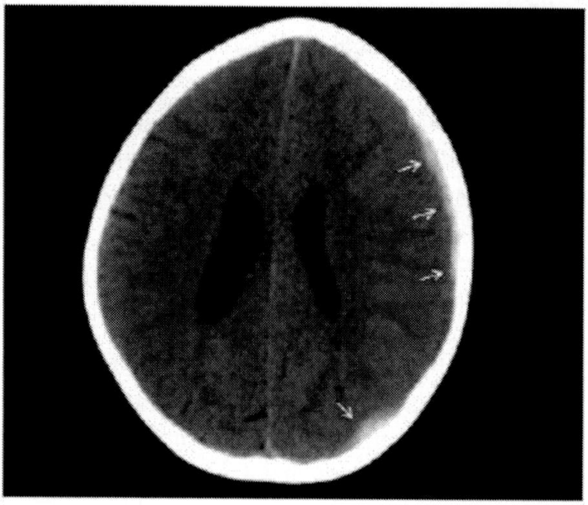

Figure 4. CT scan without contrast. Hyperdense extra-axial collection of concave morphology that spans the parieto-occipital left fossa. Corresponds to an acute subdural hematoma.

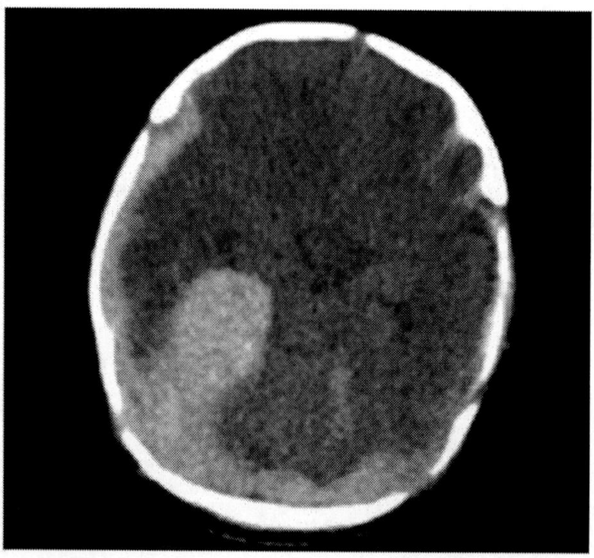

Figure 5. CT scan without contrast. Acute subdural hematoma that extends the sickle, the right convexity, the posterior fossa and tentorium, where it reaches its maximum diameter. The mass effect produces effacement of the grooves.

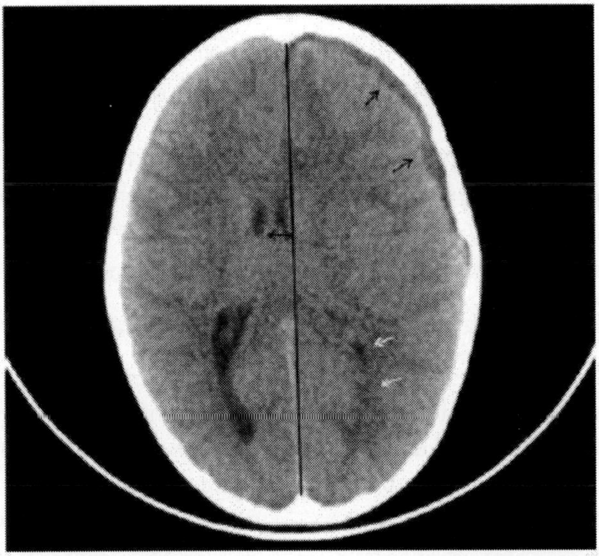

Figure 6. CT scan without contrast. Extraaxial collection of semilunar morphology, hypodense, corresponding with left frontoparietal subacute subdural hematoma (black arrows). For the mass effect determines a contralateral shift of the midline or subfalcine herniation (double black arrow) and compresses the occipital horn of left lateral ventricle (white arrows).

In patients with suspected physical abuse should be done also an **ophthalmic fundus** to rule out the presence of retinal hemorrhages. This may be delayed until the patient is stable.

In recent years it has been suggested the utility of **serum and cerebrospinal fluid markers** as *neuron-specific enolase* and *myelin-basic protein*, which could rise up in inflicted injuries and remained in normal values in accidentals [18]. If confirmed, it could be used as a screening tool in suspected cases.

Suspected cases of physical abuse should be immediately reported to the authorities. In almost all developed countries there is a multidisciplinary team responsible for managing these situations. It must also be put under protection of patients and other children living together at home, if necessary [24].

3.5.3. Treatment of Subdural Hematoma

All patients with a Glasgow <12 will benefit from an evaluation by a neurosurgeon.

Management of subdural hematoma is often more conservative than the epidural's. There is not clear surgery indication. Some possible indications of surgical management should be [4]:

- Hematoma thicker than 10 mm or midline shift > 5 mm
- Hematoma of <10 mm or midline shift <5 mm if also associated:
- Drop of ≥ 2 points on the GCS from admission
- and / or asymmetric or mydriatic pupils unresponsive
- and / or ICP> 20 mmHg

In subdural hematomas, performing prompt surgery is not associated with good outcome so clearly as in the epidural because of the possibility of associated parenchymal damage [17]. However, lack of recovery of consciousness after traumatic brain injury in a patient with subdural hematoma is an indication for immediate surgery, because of the possibility of underlying injury [24].

Patients with subdural hematomas with minimal symptoms (vomiting or irritability,without depressed level of consciousness nor focal signs) with liquified hematoma can be treated by percutaneous subdural puncture[4]. Sometimes it is necessary to place a subdural-peritoneal shunt, especially in cases where subdural hematoma becomes chronic [23].

If the hematoma requires surgical drainage, craniotomy is recommended.

Those patients in which non-surgical management is choosn should be admitted for close observation. A intracranial pressure monitor should be placed in all patients with subdural hematoma and GCS <9 [23]. Head CT should be done within 24 hours of admission, or sooner if there is a clinical worsening.

3.6. Follow-Up and Outcome

All patients with subdural hematomas should be followed for months with image tests, because sometimes they can develop a chronic subdural hematoma or a subdural hygroma. Generally most subdural hematomas are showing signs of resolution in 4-6 weeks.

The presence of a deceleration in the growth of head circumference or intraparenchymal brain abnormalities in the first 3 months after injury are associated with poor neurodevelopmental outcome at short and long term [17].

In infants a fairly reliable method of follow-up is measuring the head perimeter [23].

Studies show an intellectual development deficit in patients who have suffered a traumatic brain injury and associated subdural hematoma in childhood. Because these deficits are mostly indicative of frontal lobe dysfunction, and this lobe develops during late childhood and adolescence, is recommended monitoring these pacients during years [17].

Children with non-accidental head injury have poor prognosis at short term, with an associated mortality between 11 and 36%. In survivors, morbidity is common, ranging from learning disabilities to severe cognitive and physical disabilities in nearly two thirds of the pacients [17].

In patients with traumatic subdural hematoma prognosis depends more on underlying brain injury than the size of the hematoma. However, the prognosis is much better in accidental hematomas than in inflicted ones. This explains for two main reasons. One is the older age of patients with accidental injuries, and the other, the different mechanism of injury and frequent delays in seeking care in non-accidentals [17].

In infants with subdural hematomas associated with delivery, prognosis is good, and most are resolved within four weeks, without sequelae.

4. Subarachnoid Hemorrhage

4.1. Introduction

The subarachnoid space separates the arachnoid membrane of the pia mater, and communicates with the brain ventricles. It is filled with cerebrospinal fluid, like cerebral ventricles. Vascularization comes from both internal carotid arteries.

4.2. Etiology

Subarachnoid hematomas are the accumulation of blood in this space. These can be primary or secondary. The primaries are those in which there is only blood in the subarachnoid space and may be due to [16]:

- In newborns, delivery trauma, producing traction and secondarily, laceration of blood vessels that run through the subarachnoid space.

- In preterm infants, although it is more common than in the term neonate, pathophysiology is not well known. Is believed to be due to circulatory events related to prematurity.
- In older children and adolescents,to rupture of middle cerebral artery aneurysms and vessel of arachnoid cysts walls, usually because of minor head injuries. A typical location of the subarachnoid hematomas secondary to trauma is in the interpeduncular cistern or Silvio cissure [11].

Secondaries are produced by extension of bleeding from any other location within the skull.

4.3. Symptomatology

In neonates are often asymptomatic. When there are symptoms, it resembles to the subdural hematomas. The child may have seizures. Generally the level of consciousness between attacks is normal, although some patients may associate depressed level of conscience [16]. Sometimes the blood can be mixed with CSF, circulating throughout the brain and spinal cord, and producing meningeal irritation.

Hydrocephalus can occur from obstruction of CSF circulation, but this happens rarely [25].

In older children and adolescents, the most common symptom is headache, sometimes associated with vomiting, syncope, meningism and / or photophobia [4]. In some ocassions main symptom is a decreased level of consciousness, although it usually recovers later.

4.5. Laboratory and Image Tests

The main diagnostic test in suspected subarachnoid hemorrhage is a **head CT**. It helps to locate the hematoma and to determine its size. Hyperdense blood is usually seen in the basal cisterns or subarachnoid spaces. In hematomas secondary to rupture of an aneurysm, the location could indicate the site of aneurysm [11]. In these cases should be indicate performing an **angio-CT scan** with contrast.

The rapid dilution of the blood in the CSF may difficult detection of subarachnoid hematoma by **MRI**.

Transfontanelar ultrasound is few sensitive to detect this kind of hematoma.

Most sensitive test for detection of subarachnoid hematoma would be performing a **lumbar puncture**, in which could find [4]:

- Increased CSF output pressure
- Xanthochromic and bloody fluid, which subsequently clarified.
- RBC count> 100,000 cells/mm^3
- Increased proteins level in CSF
- CSF glucose level normal or impaired

However, this test should not be performed if there are signs of intracranial hypertension.

4.6. Treatment

Non-surgical management is usually performed in an intensive care unit, with adequate hydric input (it is important to maintain adequate blood pressure for assureing a good cerebral perfusion pressure), oxygenation and sedation (use of morphine generally will be necessary). Use of antiepileptic drugs prophylactically is controversial, but currently is not indicated. The main complications to be monitored should be [4]:

- *Intracranial hypertension* (see *treatment of epidural hematoma*)
- *Syndrome of inadequate ADH secretion:* frequent monitoring of ions in blood must be done, and ensure adequate intake of sodium. No water restriction must be made by the risk of hypotension.
- *Rebleeding:* assessing the use of antifibrinolytic drugs (aminocaproic acid) or selective embolization of the bleeding.
- *Hydrocephalus:* caused by obstruction of CSF circulation. Sometimes it requires a ventriculostomy to relieve the increased pressure.

4.7. Follow-Up and Outcome

Prognosis of subarachnoid hematomas in infants is usually good. In older patients with hematomas secondary to ruptured aneurysms or arteriovenous malformations, the main prognostic factors are prompt medical care and neurological status prior to care.

5. Intraventricular Hemorrhage

It is a disease almost exclusive of preterm infants, and often secondary to hypoxic-ischemic insult in the perinatal period. Germinal matrix is a region very sensitive to hypotension and hypoperfusion, and hemorrhage commonly occur at this point after an asphyxictic event. Factors that increase the risk of this disease, mainly an increase in cerebral perfusion pressure and increased cerebral blood flow. Other factors would be low weight at birth, maternal chorioamnionitis, antenatal steroid use for fetal lung maturity, maternal coagulopathy or abuse of substances such as cocaine.

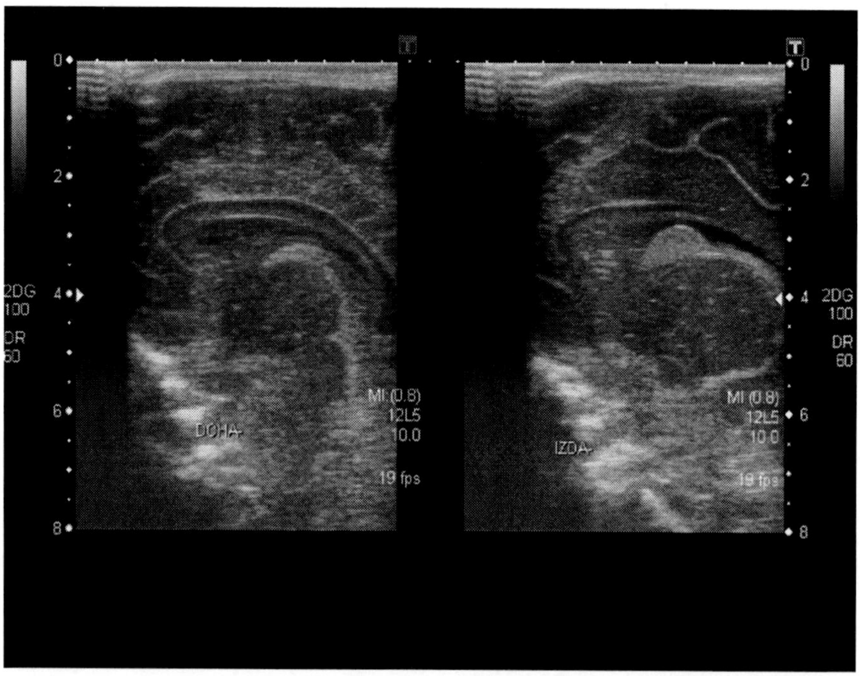

Figure 7. Transfontanelar ultrasound, sagittal images. Hyperechoic nodule in the left thalamus-caudate sulcus consistent with acute hemorrhage of the germinal matrix.

Table 2. Grading of intraventricular hemorrhage

Grado	Descripción
I	subependimal
II	IVH without ventricular dilatation
III	IVH with ventricular dilatation
IV	IVH with parenchymal hemorrhage

Most intraventricular hemorrages occur in two period. A vast majority occur in the first 12 hours of life, and many others between 3 and 4 days of life.

Many of these hemorrhages are asymptomatic and are discovered by chance when performing an ultrasound transfontanelar control. When symptomatic, it is seen a decrease in tone, the presence of apnea or bradycardia or the presence of seizures, although the latter often are subclinical [4].

Diagnosis is made by transfontanelar ultrasound [11] (Figure 7), which also determines the extent of bleeding (Table 2). In doubtful cases a head CT or MRI can be done.

Treatment is supportive, treating the complications that may arise. In cases where hydrocephalus occurs, it may require placement of an intraventricular drainage catheter.

Prognosis for these patients depends on the size of the hemorrhage, as well as gestational age and associated pathology. In large hemorrhages often develop hydrocephalia *ex-vacuo*, because of the loss of brain tissue, without an increase in ICP.

References

[1] Kahle W, Leonhardt H, Platzer w. Atlas de anatomía para estudiantes y médicos. *Tomo 3: sistema nervioso y órganos de los sentidos. 5ª ed.* Barcelona: Ediciones Omega; 1999.

[2] Ahn ES, Proctor MR. Intracranial epidural hematoma in children: Epidemiology, anatomy and pathophysiology. Available at: *http://www.uptodate.com/contents/intracranial-epidural-hematoma-in-children-epidemiology-anatomy-and-pathophysiology?source=search_result&selectedTitle=3%7E50*

[3] Case ME. Accidental traumatic head injury in infants and young children. *Brain Pathol.* 2008 Oct;18(4):583-9
[4] Greenberg MS. *Handbook of Neurosurgery.* 7 ed. New York:. Thieme Medical Publishers; 2006
[5] Orliaguet GA, Meyer PG, Baugnon T. Management of critically ill children with traumatic brain injury. *Paediatr Anaesth.* 2008 Jun;18(6):455-61.
[6] Guía manejo del paciente politraumatizado SEUP. Available at: *http://www.saludaliamedica.com/Med/protocolos/seup/SEUP_politrauma/SEUP_politraumaABCDE.htm*
[7] Manrique Martínez I, Alcalá Minagorre PJ. Manejo del traumatismo cranial pediátrico. Protocolos diagnósticos-terapéuticos de Urgencias Pediátricas SEUP-AEP. Available at: *http://www.aeped.es/sites/default/files/documentos/manejo_del_traumatismo_craneal_pediatrico.pdf*
[8] Vavilala MS, Bowen A, Lam AM, Uffman JC, Powell J, Winn HR et al. Blood pressure and outcome after severe pediatric traumatic brain injury. *J Trauma.* 2003 Dec;55(6): 1039-44
[9] Trenchs V, Curcoy A, Castillo M, Badosa J, Luaces C, Pou J et al. Minor head trauma and linear skull fracture in infants: cranial ultrasound or computer tomography?. *Eur J Emerg Med.* 2009 Jun;16(3):150-2
[10] Traboild F, Meyer PG, Blanot S, Carli PA, orliaguet GA. The prognostic value of transcranial Doppler studies in children with moderate and severe head injury. *Intensive Care Med.* 2004 Jan;30(1):108-12.
[11] Huisman TA. Intracraneal hemorrhage: ultrasound, CT and MRI findings. *Eur Radiol.* 2005 Mar;15(3):434-40.
[12] Ucar T, Akyuz M, Kazan S, Tuncer R. Role of decompressive surgery in the management of severe head injuries: prognostic factors and patient selection. *J Neurotrauma.* 2005 nov;22(11):1311-8
[13] Suarez EP, González AS, Diaz CP, Salido Ag, de Azagra Garde AM, Flores JC. Decompressive craniectomy in 14 children with severe head injury: clinical results with long-term follow-up and review of the literature. *J Trauma.* 2011 Jul;71(1):133-40
[14] Ahn ES, Proctor MR. Intracranial epidural hematoma in children: Clinical features, evaluation, and management. Available at: *http://www.uptodate.com/contents/intracranial-epidural-hematoma-in-children-clinical-features-evaluation-and-management?source=search_result&selectedTitle=2%7E50*

[15] Mack J, Squier W, Eastman JT. Anatomy and development of the meninges: implications for subdural collections and CSF circulation. *Pediatr Radiol.* 2009 Mar;39(3):200-10
[16] Barker S. Subdural and primary subarachnoid hemorrhages: a case study. *Neonatal Netw.* 2007 May-jun;26(3):143-51
[17] Jayawant S, Parr J. Outcome following subdural haemorrhages in infancy. *Arch Dis Child.* 2007 Apr;92(4):343-7.
[18] Berger RP, Dulani T, Adelson D, Leventhal JM, Richichi R, Kochanek PM. Identification of inflicted traumatic brain injury in well-appearing infants using serum and cerebrospinal markers: a possible screening tool. *Pediatrics.* 2006 Feb;11782):325-32.
[19] Salomao JF, Leibinger RD, Lima YM. Chronic subdural hematoma as a complication of ventriculoperitoneal shunts. *Arq Neuropsiquiatr.* 1990 Jun;48(2):217-24
[20] Sridhar K, Venkateswara PG, Ramakrishnaiah S, Iyer V. Posttraumatic retroclival acute subdural hematoma: report of two cases and review of literature. *Neurol India.* 2010 Nov-Dec;58(6):945-8
[21] Velasco Zúñiga R, Fernández Arribas JL, Puente Montes S, Gutiérrez Abad C. Post-traumatic subdural haematoma associated with an arachnoid cyst. *An Pediatr* (Barc). 2011 Mar 2 [Epub ahead of print]
[22] Pou I Fernandez J. Maltrato infantil. Actuación en urgencias. Protocolos diagnósticos-terapéuticos de Urgencias Pediátricas SEUP-AEP. Available at: *http://www.aeped.es/sites/default/files/documentos/maltrato_infantil._actuacion_en_urgencias.pdf*
[23] Proctor MR. Intracranial subdural hematoma in children: Clinical features, evaluation, and management. Available at: *http://www.uptodate.com/contents/intracranial-subdural-hematoma-in-children-clinical-features-evaluation-and-management?source=search_result&selectedTitle=16%7E50*
[24] Atabaki SM. Pediatric head injury. *Pediatr Rev.* 2007 Jun;28(6):215-24
[25] Alfonso I, Andrade EO, Luzondo RJ, Diaz-Arca G, PApazian O. Cerebrovascular accidents in full-term newborn infants. *Rev Neurol.* 2006 Apr 10;42 Suppl 3:S17-22.

In: Hematomas: Types, Treatments ... ISBN: 978-1-61942-385-5
Editors: M.F.G.Salazar...pp. 171-178

Chapter VI

Massive Retroperitoneal Hematoma Following Vaginal Correction of Vault Prolapse

Alberto López García*[*]*, Luis Vázquez Illanes and Talal Diab Halawa
Servicio De Obstetricia Y Ginecología.
Hospital Lucus Augusti. Lugo, Spain

Abstract

We wish to describe an acute case of the formation of an uncommonly large hematoma in the retroperitoneal following a vaginal intervention. This is a case report of a 72 year-old hypertensive patient on treatment with enoxaparin, among other medication, for several days before being admitted to hospital. She undergoes surgery for a cystorectocele with vaginal vault prolapse, using the vaginal way. After 36 hours she presents intense low back pain with deteriorated general state of health. The C.T. scan reveals a large hematoma approximately 16 centimeters in size with active bleeding in abdominal cavity. The case is presented for discussion and we review any medical literature concerning the appearance of this complication following gynecological

[*] Address: Alberto López García Servicio de Obstetricia y Ginecología. Hospital Lucus Augusti, San Cibrao s/n, Lugo, SPAIN, e-mail: alberto.lopez.garcia@sergas.es

interventions in patients treated with enoxparin In spite of its low prevalence following gynecological surgeries, a retroperitoneal hematoma may turn into an extremely serious complication. For this reason, the likelihood of a similar situation occurring is to be kept in mind in certain circumstances. The literature concerning the afore-mentioned complication in gynecological vaginal interventions is scarce with only rare publications of individual cases. Nevertheless, in these past years a certain number of cases related to retroperitoneal hematoma occurring spontaneously in patients being treated with enoxoparin have been published. The patients affected are fundamentally elderly, with heart disease and relative deterioration of their renal function. We were unable to discover the statistical frequency of this complication following vaginal surgery, however it is believed to be rather uncommon. In any case we consider it of interest that other specialists be aware of the possibility of its occurrence considering the seriousness of the situation.

Keywords: vaginal surgery, vaginal vault prolapse, retroperitoneal hematoma.

Case Report

A 72 year-old woman G3P3 who suffers from hypertension, heart disease with dilation of ascending aorta, diabetes mellitus(type 2) and chronic broncopathy is on oral treatment with *nifedipin*, 60 mg./day (antihypertensive, calcium antagonist), *fosinopril* 20 mg./day (angiotensin converting enzyme inhibitor, antihypertensive), acetylsalicylic acid 150 mg./ day (anticoagulant) and acetylcysteine 600 mg. /day (mucolytic agent). Previous surgeries of patient include a total hysterectomy as well as a bilateral oophorectomy performed 26 years before for uterine myoma and uterine hemorrhage.

The gynecological procedure to be described consists of a vaginal vault prolapse, cystocele grade 3 and a *rectoenterocele grade 1 and 2*, symptomatic. A right inguinal hernia was also diagnosed. After a favourable evaluation by the department of anesthesia, it was decided that the correction of the prolapse be performed by the department of gynecology while the inguinal herniaplasty was to be carried out by the department of general surgery during the same intervention. Treatment with acetylsalicylic acid was substituted by a low - molecular-weight heparin (enoxaparin, 60 mg./ 6000IU /0,6 ml. five days before the intervention. The vaginal surgical procedure consisted of correction using vaginal way. First we made an incision in the vagina, anterior plasty; then a dissection of the enterocele and reduction of the latter were performed as well as a posterior plasty. Redundant vagina was removed. The department of surgery carried out the inguinal hernioplasty surturing a wire mesh for reenforcement. The patient suffered a difficult postoperative period. After 36 hours she experienced severe low back pain, in spite of intravenous analgesia as demanded by protocol, and a progressive deterioration of general state of health. An urgent ultrasound diagnosis and blood analysis were requested. The radiology department decided to perform a computerized tomographic scan (see images 1 to 4).

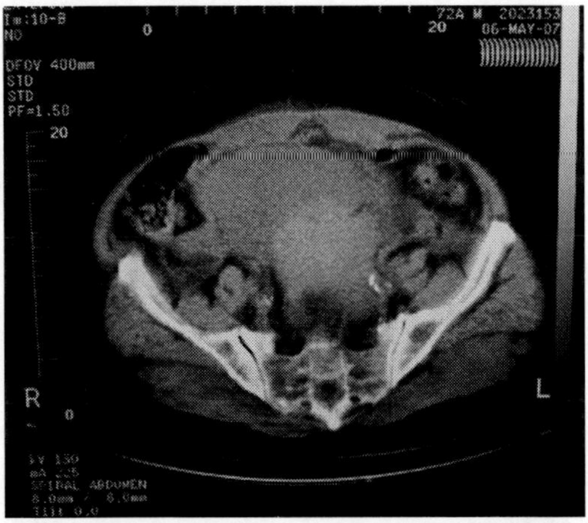

Image 1. Retroperitoneal Haematoma.

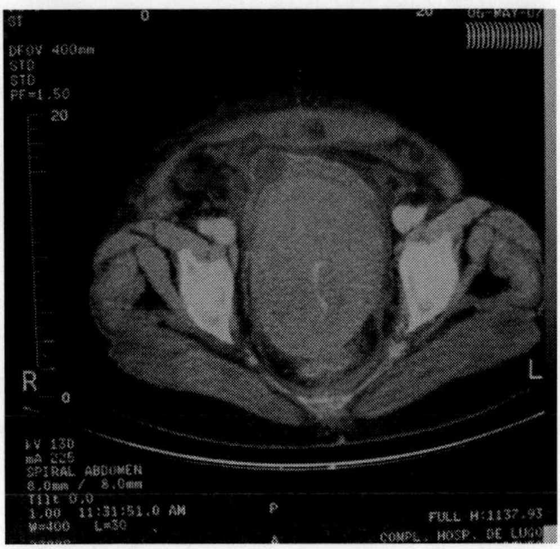

Image 2. Retroperitoneal Haematoma.

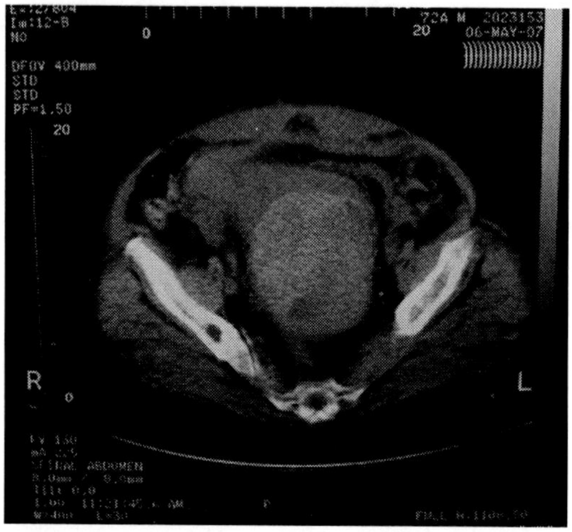

Image 3. retroperitoneal haematoma.

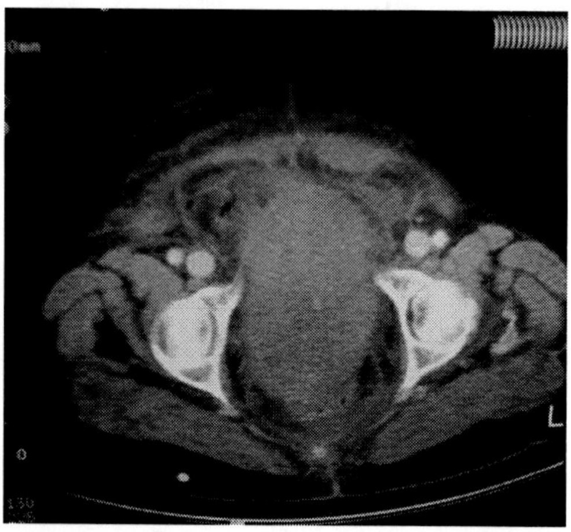

Image 4. Retroperitoneal Haematoma.

We were informed of the existence of an extremely large mass which occupied the entire pelvic region compatible to a hematoma larger than 16 cm. in size with signs of active bleeding. The blood analysis showed a loss of practically 8g./ dl. of hemaglobin and a drop of 24 units in the hematocrit count compared to preoperative levels, however platelets and blood clotting were within normal limits.

Immediately 7 units of platelet-enriched plasma were administered and a midline laparotomy is performed under general anesthesia. We observed an abdominal cavity with no signs of bleeding but with an enormous bulging retroperitoneal tumour that occupied the entire pelvis extending to the kidney vessels.

We proceeded to incise the peritoneal membrane and access the retroperitoneum through its most prominent zone. It was impossible for us to identify the anatomical structures with clarity due to the infiltration of membranes and spaces with dark coagulated blood. A roman dissection is cautiously performed reaching an elastic-like section of mass adhered to the posterior wall which is incided producing an abundant amount of blood clotting and dark blood.

Confronted with the impossibility of locating with precision the bleeding point, we decided to fill the space of the excised tumour with absorbable hemostats (Surgice [l]), leaving the retroperitoneum with an opening into the abdominal cavity and placing surgical drains with aspiration system. Intravenous antibiotic treatment is administered. The patient presented a satisfactory postoperative period with evident recovery and disappearance of low back pain.

Discussion

Based on the review of medical literature concerning retroperitoneal hematoma as a complication resulting from a gynecological intervention via vagina, we are able to affirm that hardly any data or statistics with reference to case frequency were available; thus we assumed that the process is rather uncommon or even rare. Indeed the cases found were scarce and published many years back. One case cited occurred following a vaginal hysterectomy [1] and another after a cold knife conization [2]. Given the rarity of the problem, it is difficult to conclude that factors deriving from the surgery or the patient herself would predispose her to suffer said complication.

In obstetrics we came upon cases concerning retroperitoneal hematomas during puerperium. This complication has been related to a spontaneous rupture of an ovarian artery . Also intra- and retroperitoneal haemorrhage have been described to occur for the same reason on the second day of puerperium [3,4].

Another possible cause for retroperitoneal hematomas could result from complications in laparoscopy [5,6], due to the insertion of blind trocars. There also exists evidence of retroperitoneal haemorrhaging complications induced by oocyte retrieval for in vitro fertilization [7].

Recently the appearance of several cases of retroperitoneal bleeding in patients treated with enoxparin have been reported [8-14]. According to papers published the spontaneous retroperitoneal hematomas occurred in patients admitted to critical units after preoperative therapeutical dosage of enoxaparin, alone or associated to other anticoagulants/ antiagreggants. These patients are usually elderly, affected by acute coronary syndrome, peripheral thrombosis or other pathologies that justify anticoagulation. Frequently renal failure may also be associated to these patients, which in turn would complicate the elimination of heparin.

We know that the risk of hemorrhage is unlikely with the use of low-molecular-weight heparin, but it increases in cases of heart disease, renal or hepatic insufficiency and in patients over 60. Ernits and cols.[8] suggest the median frequency of the appearance of hematoma is after 5 days of enoxaparin therapy at therapeutic doses (1 mg./ kg./ 12 h.), in patients with risk factors (advanced age, kidney deterioration, receiving concomitant treatment which affects hemostasis). They propose being alert to the major symptoms of hemorrhaging and monitorizing the anti-factor Xa in high risk patients.

We have reported a case of massive retroperitoneal hematoma following the repair of a vaginal vault prolapse by vaginal surgery. In our experience the patient presented intense progressive low back pain several hours after surgery, followed by evident deterioration of her general state of health. This leads us to believe that the pain was a consequence of the growth of the hematoma, which gradually infiltrated the retroperitoneum. Progressively the increase in the volume of blood retained began to alter the patient's vital constants.

Evidently the images (C.T.scan and ultrasound) were of great assistance in reaching a diagnosis. As far as the treatment is concerned, it seems obvious that in cases of hematomas in evolution and shock patients, we should intervene actively. In our case the patient was urgently submitted to surgery, but we ignore whether radiologic embolization might be of interest, or even if it would be justifiable expectant management. Some colleagues might even propose treatment with recombinant activated factor VII [14].

An urgent surgical intervention in the retroperitoneal space may be extremely complicated, and even more so if the coagulated blood infiltrates and increases the pressure and wall tension within the cavity, consequently impeding a clear identification of anatomical structures. In our case we managed to drain a great number of blood clots. Although we did not manage to identify the blood vessel or vessels causing the hematoma in order to perform a hemostasis, we were more than happy to fill the evacuated cavity with reabsorbable Surgicel ®.

References

[1] Lev-Gur M, Patel S, Greston WM, McGill F. Pararenal hematoma as a complication of vaginal hysterectomy. A case report. *J. Reprod. Med.* 1987 Jan; 32(1):68-71.

[2] Brown CF, Mashini IS, Turner WA, Gallup DG. Retroperitoneal hematoma: an unusual complication of cold knife conization of the cervix. *Obstet. Gynecol.* 1986 Sep; 68(3 Suppl):66S-67S.

[3] Burnett RA, Carfrae DC. Spontaneus rupture of ovarian artery aneurysm in the puerperium. Two case reports and review of the literature. *Br. J. Obstet. Gynaecol.* 1976 Sep; 83(9):744-50.

[4] Banas T, Boryczko M, Durzynska-Urbaniec J. Intraperitoneal hemorrhage due to the rupture of right ovarian artery in the second day of puerperium. *Ginekol. Pol.* 2004 Sep; 75(9):729-32.

[5] Zweigel D, Thiele H, Schworm HD. Injuries of large vessels caused by laparoscopy. *Zentralbl Gynakol.* 1987; 109(10):673-8.

[6] Leron E, Piura B, Ohana E, Mazor M. Delayed recognition of major vascular injury during laparoscopy. *Eur. J. Obstet. Gynecol. Reprod. Biol.* 1998 Jul; 79(1):91-3.

[7] Azem F, Wolf Y, Botchan A, Amit A, Lessing JB, Kluger Y. Massive retroperitoneal bleeding: a complication of transvaginal ultrasonography-guided oocyte retrieval for in vitro fertilization-embryo transfer. *Fertil Steril,* 2000 Aug; 74(2):405-6.

[8] Ernits M, Mohan PS, Fares LG 2nd, Hardy H 3rd. A retroperitoneal bleed induced by enoxaparin theraphy. *Am. Surg.* 2005 May; 71 (5):430-3.

[9] Topgul K, Uzum O, Anadol AZ, Gok A. Surgical management of enoxaparin- and/or warfarin-induced massive retroperitoneal bleeding: report of a case and review of the literature. *South Med. J.* 2005 Jan; 98(1):104-6.

[10] Mrug M, Mishra PV, Lusane HC, Cunningham JM, Alpert MA. Hemothorax and retroperitoneal hematoma after anticoagulation with enoxaparin. *South Med. J.* 2002 Aug;95(8):936-8.

[11] Chan-Tack KM. Fatal spontaneous retroperitoneal hematoma secondary to enoxaparin. *South Med. J.* 2003 Jan; 96(1):58-60.

[12] Dabney A, Bastani B. Enoxaparin-associated severe retroperitoneal bleeding and abdominal compartment syndrome: a report of two cases. *Intensive. Care. Med.* 2001 Dec; 27(12):1954-7. Epub 2001 Nov 10.

[13] Gomez de la Torre R, Milla Crespo A, Cadenas F, Fernandez Bustamante J, Vazquez Castanon M. Spontaneus retroperitoneal hematoma induced by enoxaparin to therapeutic dose. *An Med. Interna.* 2003 Jul; 20(7):386-7.

[14] Cherfan A, Arabi Y, Askar AA, Shimemeri AA. Recombinant Activated Factor VII Treatment of Retroperitoneal Hematoma in a Patient with Renal Failure Receiving Enoxaparin and Clopidrogrel. *Pharmacotherapy.* 2007 May; 27 (5):755-9.

In: Hematomas: Types, Treatments ... ISBN: 978-1-61942-385-5
Editors: M.F.G.Salazar...pp. 179-196

Chapter VII

Retropharyngeal Hematoma

Tun-Yen Hsu*

Department of Otolaryngology, E-DA Hospital / I-Shou University, 1, Yi-Da Road,Jiau-shu Tsuen, Yan-chau Shiang, Kaohsiung County, Taiwan, R.O.C.

Abstract

Retropharyngeal hematoma is an uncommon entity of disease of pharynx. A variety of causes are known including direct neck trauma, whiplash injury, foreign body ingestion, deep neck infection, metastatic carcinoma, anticoagulant drugs, coughing, sneezing, straining, or even spontaneous bleeding. Diagnosis can often be inferred from history but exploration may be required for confirmation. Due to pharyngeal wall swelling, it wound cause sore throat, dysphonia, dysphagia or even dyspnea while airway compromise. Physical examination may reveal stridor. In some severe cases, subcutaneous bruising over neck and anterior chest may be found. Narrowing of the pharynx can be detected simply by neck soft tissue lateral view X-ray or by endoscopic examination. Computed tomography (CT) scan or Magnetic Resonance Imaging (MRI) examination should also be necessary because the hematoma may involve inferiorly to the mediastinum causing anterior displacement of trachea or esophagus which complicate management

* Corresponding author: E-mail: dunyen@yahoo.com.tw, ed102345@edah.org.tw; Tel: +886-7-6150011-2970; Fax: +886-7-6150913.

strategy. Securing the airway is the most crucial. In traumatic cases, cervical spine immobilization is also important. Surgical evacuation of a retropharyngeal hematoma can be necessary when the hematoma is large, breathing inadequate or conservative management unsuccessful. Specific management against the possible specific cause should also be taken.

Introduction

Disease involving the retropharyngeal area is relatively uncommon. The retropharyngeal area is of potential spaces between pharyngeal wall and vertebrae which is composed of fatty tissue and lymph nodes. Once there is space occupying lesion in these spaces, the confining fascias will be distended anteriorly and compromise the upper as well as lower aerodigestive tracts. Therefore, dyspnea, dysphagia, sore throat or odynophagia will commence. Undoubtedly, if the volume of the space occupying lesion is so big that complete obstruction of the airway occurs, emergent airway establishment is required. The above mentioned space occupying lesion can be abscess, hematoma, enlarged lymph node or even tumor [1]. Hematoma means an abnormal localized collection of blood which is usually situated within an organ or a soft tissue space. Although retropharyngeal hematoma is an uncommon disease, the life threatening condition may sometimes be overlooked as ordinary upper respiratory tract inflammation or infection [2]. Therefore, it is worthwhile comprehensively understanding the disease.

Anatomy

There are three anatomical spaces identified between the pharyngeal wall and vertebra. The first one is retropharyngeal space which is also named posterior visceral space, is between visceral fascia and alar fascia, extending from the skull base to T4. The second one is danger space which is between alar fascia and prevertebral fascia, extending from the skull base to the diaphragm. The third one is prevertebral space which is between the prevertebral fascia and the anterior ligament of the vertebral column. The danger space provides a direct pathway for head and neck infections to spread into the posterior mediastinum. Neither the retropharyngeal space nor the danger space can be demonstrated in normal individual [1,3,4].

Etiology

Many possible causes of retropharyngeal hematoma were reported.

Neck Trauma

It is undoubtedly that neck trauma is one common cause of retropharyngeal hematoma [5,6,7,8]. The so-called trauma ranged from mild or blunt neck jolt [9,10,11,12,13,14,15], occipital trauma or occipital condyle fracture [16,17,18], whiplash injury [19], airbag injury [20], to many other various kinds of cervical trauma with or without cervical spine fracture [6,21,22,23,24,26,27,28,29,30,31,32,33,34,35, 36,37]. Major trauma may reasonably induce hematoma formation but how about minor blunt trauma? O'Neill explained that this injury was caused by flexion followed by hyperextension of the cervical spine [12,38]. It was believed that formation of hematoma in cases of cervical spine trauma is from tearing of the longus colli muscles along the anterior aspect of the vertebral bodies [19]. Penning explained the injury wound cause extensive anterior ligamentous damage with rupture of larger blood vessels covering the anterior aspect of the vertebral column since the ligaments themselves area poorly vascularized and the avulsion fracture area of insignificant sizes [21].

Hemorrhagic Diathesis

There were two kinds of hemorrhagic diathesis were associated with retropharyngeal hematoma and were reported. One was hemophilia [39,40,41] and the other was polycythemia vera (even in general it cause a thrombotic complication)[42]. Most of them were noted to have bleeding tendency and rests of them were still associated to trauma.

Anticoagulant Usage

Major bleeding episodes have been reported to occur in approximately 2-4% of patients being treated with oral anticoagulants [43]. Some of the patients using anticoagulant suffered from retropharyngeal hematoma were also attributed to trauma or other causes. Anticoagulants such as warfarin [5,43,44,45,46,47,48,49], dicumarol [50,51], heparin[44], Coumadin[20,52], acenocoumarol [53], and dipyridamol[41] were reported to be associated with retropharyngeal hematoma. Aspirin was also mentioned as a possible contributing factor because of its platelet modifying function [7,41,54,55,56,57]. In most of the cases using anticoagulants, the prothrombin time or the partial thromboplastin time were prolonged. But in some cases, the data were normal.

Neck Infection

Three cases of neck infection were associated with major bleeding and retropharyngeal hematoma formation [44,58,59]. It is not a common complication of neck infection but should be kept in mind.

Foreign Body

Three cases of foreign body were associated with retropharyngeal hematoma and were reported [60,61,62]. It is not a common complication of foreign body mis-swallowing but should also be kept in mind.

Spontaneous

Spontaneous retropharyngeal hematoma is defined if there is no obvious cause such as trauma or bleeding tendency can explain the bleeding [7,8,39,57,63,64,65].

Other Possible Causes

There are still many possible causes related to the formation of the hematoma at the retropharyngeal area: cervical arthroplasty [66], parathyroid adenoma[67,68], parathyroid cyst [69], parathyroid apoplexy [70], carotid sinus massage [71], aneurysm rupture [5,72,73], jugular vein cannulation [74], stellate ganglion block [75,76], after vomiting [77], strain [55], sneezing [5,50], coughing [24], muscle exertion[5], turn suddenly [24], after upper respiratory tract infection [40], Epstein-Barr virus [78], and an initial presentation of metastatic prostatic cancer [79].

Diagnosis

History

It is absolutely necessary to know the patient's past medical history and present illness in order to make a correct diagnosis. Because retropharyngeal hematoma is a disease affecting the upper aerodigestive tract and is acute onset, it is necessary to differentiate from some other upper aerodigestive tract emergency such as foreign body impaction, acute supraglottic laryngitis or acute epiglottitis, or deep neck infection. The common causes of retropharyngeal hematoma should be sought and even trivial trauma or minor movement should be noted. Different causes of retropharyngeal hematoma should raise different management strategies.

Symptoms

Generally, due to space-occupying hematoma formation in the retropharyngeal area including retropharyngeal space, danger space, and prevertebral space, the pharyngeal wall will bulge into the pharyngeal lumen compromising the upper as well as lower aerodigestive tracts and make the patients feel sore throat, odynophagia, dysphagia, and dyspnea. Some patients may also feel neck pain and neck stiffness and therefore are unwilling to turn their neck. If the hematoma formation involves the mediastinum, the patients will feel chest pain, too. In some cases, the velocity of the hematoma formation is slow and the presentation of the symptoms may delay [6,10]. As to the patients of neck injury, we must keep in mind of the possibility of cervical spine injury.

Physical Examination

On examination, ecchymosis may be seen at the neck area and anterior chest (Figure 1). Due to the upper aerodigestive tract compromises, the patients may have noisy, stridulous respiration. The voice may be muffled. Tachypnea or orthopnea may also be noted.

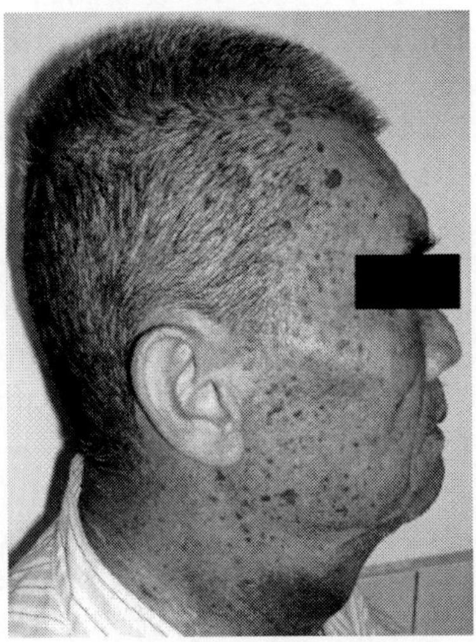

Figure 1. Ecchymosis at anterior neck area in a patient of retropharyngeal hematoma.

Endoscopic Evaluation

For detailed examination, fiberoptic scope examination is performed through nasal cavity into pharynx, and it may reveal ecchymosis at the bulging posterior pharyngeal wall (Figure 2) and the degree of the upper aerodigestive tract compromise. Saliva pooling may be found. It is highly recommended to do fiberoptic scope examination either in the initial diagnosis stage or at regular following up stage because it is neither invasive nor of radiation exposure.

Radiologic Evaluation

The most simple and non invasive way to understand the condition of pharynx is plain X-ray evaluation. Wholey et al. had reviewed 600 normal lateral neck films and it showed that in adults (480 cases), the distance from the anterior-inferior aspect of the second cervical vertebra to the posterior wall of the pharynx should be 1–7 mm (average = 3.4mm); the distance from the anterior-inferior aspect of the sixth cervical vertebra to the posterior aspect of the trachea should be 9–22 mm (average = 14 mm) In children 15 years and under (120 cases), the distance from the anterior-inferior aspect of the second cervical vertebra to the posterior wall of the pharynx should be 2–7 mm (average = 3.5mm); the distance from the anterior-inferior aspect of the sixth cervical vertebra to the posterior aspect of the trachea should be 5–14 mm (average = 7.9 mm)[80]. Any thickness of correspondent area is larger than the normal value mentioned above should raise the suspicion of retropharyngeal disease (Figure 3). Plain X-ray evaluation should include chest X-ray film as well as neck soft tissue film because the hematoma may involve the mediastinum (Figure 4).

In the modern time, CT is widely available in many hospitals. CT can actually provide us anatomical change and the extension of the retropharyngeal hematoma more than plain X-ray in short time. We can know exactly the critical obstruction area in patients of retropharyngeal hematoma presenting dyspnea. However, the CT image of the retropharyngeal hematoma is not always so specific and may not aid us so much in making differential diagnosis (Figure 5).

MRI is superior to CT in the diagnosis of retropharyngeal hematoma. MRI is sensitive to blood products in different stages of evolution because of the paramagnetic signal properties of the blood products which change over the time depending on their dominant component (acute deoxyhemoglobin, subacute intra- or extreacellular methemoglobin, and chronic hemichromes) [77]. The diagnosis of hematoma can be made as early as a few hours after the acute event, when hyperintensity seen on both T1- and T2- weighted sequenced [81]. However, in contrary to CT, MRI is less available and requires more patient cooperation. Patients with retropharyngeal hematoma may be agitated for dyspnea and therefore may not be suitable for MRI evaluation [77].

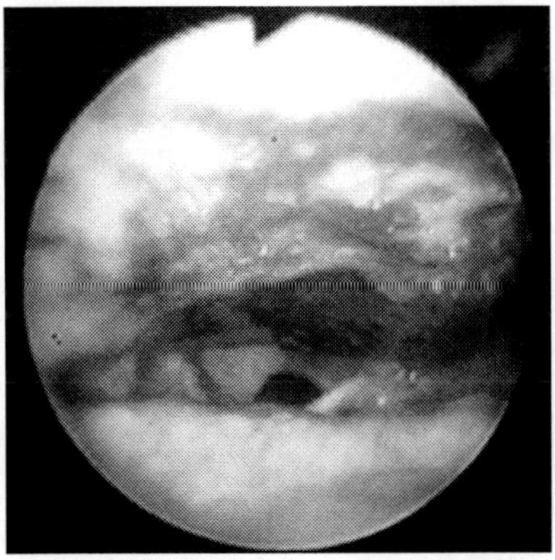

Figure 2. Ecchymosis at the bulging posterior pharyngeal wall in a patient of retropharyngeal hematoma.

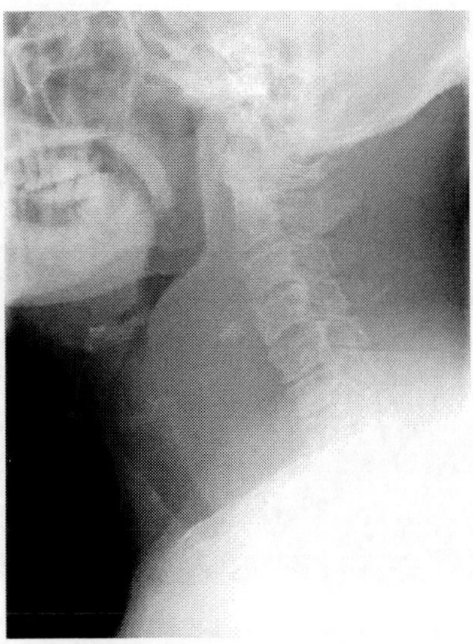

Figure 3. Abnormally increased thickness of the retropharyngeal area in a patient of retropharyngeal hematoma.

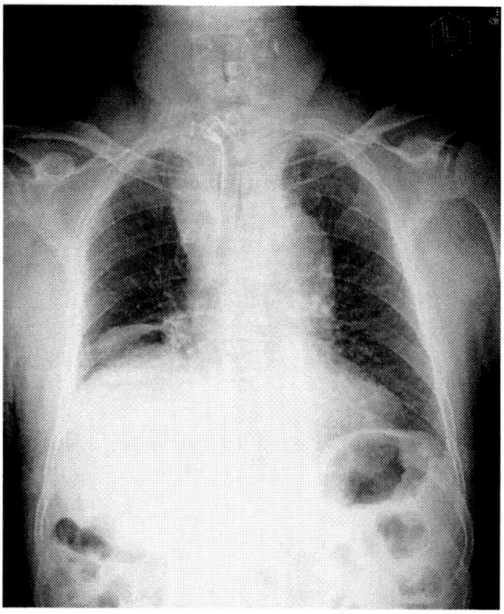

Figure 4. Widened mediastinum implying hematoma involving mediastinum in a patient of retropharyngeal hematoma.

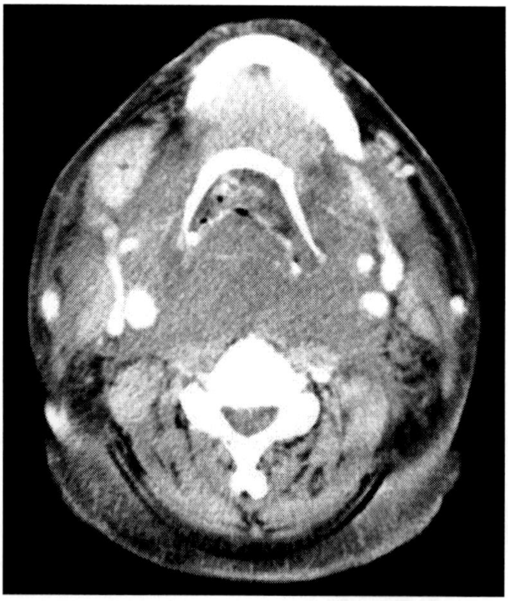

Figure 5. Mildly heterogeneously enhanced retropharyngeal swelling in a patient of retropharyngeal hematoma.

Angiography study is also of value in understanding the possible bleeder especially while hematoma is extensive and large vessels or their branches rupture is suspected [35].

Capps Triads

Capps had proposed a triad of tracheal and esophageal compression, ventral tracheal displacement on lateral cervical X-ray film and the subsequent appearance of subcutaneous bruising in the anterior neck and upper thorax which can be seen in the patients of retropharyngeal hematoma [82,83]. The triads can facilitate the diagnosis over retropharyngeal and mediastinum hematoma.

Laboratory Test

While facing the retropharyngeal hematoma, we should focus on those laboratory tests related to hemostasis, such as platelet count, prothrombin time, activated partial thromboplastin time or even bleeding time. Those who have history of anticoagulant usage are not necessary to have abnormal laboratory result. It is also necessary to pay attention to white blood cell count to help us in the differentiate infection from pure hematoma formation. Hemoglobin level and hematocrit level should also be checked to confirm whether the bleeding is severe enough to make patient anemic. Poor liver function is associated with bleeding tendency and therefore liver function test including GOT(Glutamate Oxaloacetate Transaminase), GPT(Glutamic Pyruvic Transaminase), γGT(γ- Glutamyl Transpeptidase), total bilirubin, direct bilirubin should also be performed and sonographic examination should be optionally performed if liver cirrhosis or splenomegaly are suspected.

In general, unless a typical history of possible causes mentioned above such as obvious trauma, clinical diagnosis of retropharyngeal hematoma may be difficult. Usually, while facing acute onset of retropharyngeal swelling, an initial impression is either infection or tumor.

Management

It is undoubtedly paramount to pay attention to the airway. Dyspnea may be noted immediately after trauma or may be delayed in presentation even trauma is the cause of bleeding [14]. Therefore, keeping close observation is the key of management and oxygen support is absolutely given if dyspnea is noted. If ventilation is not adequate, establish a secure airway is necessary.

The way to secure the airway is just like that in usual condition: either placement of endotracheal tube or tracheotomy. However, placement of endotracheal tube via oral cavity or nasal cavity may cause further pharyngeal wall trauma and may lead to bleeding into aerodigestive tract [6,38]. If intubation is still required, an anesthesiologist using fiberscope intubation technique is highly suggested and emergent tracheotomy or cricothyroidotomy should be available.

In addition, it is also necessary to know whether anemia occurs and makes patients dizziness. Blood transfusion may be required.

Conservative management with aspiration, observation, or medication for bleeding tendency such as Vitamin K support could be performed in minor cases. Surgical evacuation of a retropharyngeal hematoma may be necessary when the hematoma is large, breathing inadequate or conservative management unsuccessful [2].

In fact, except obvious trauma related retropharyngeal hematoma, exploration is often necessary because most of the cases of retropharyngeal hematoma are always impressed as infection or tumor initially. Only operation findings and pathological study can prove it and then other specific management against the possible specific cause should be taken accordingly.

Theoretically and generally, the way to stop bleeding is locating the bleeder followed by compression, cauterization, or ligation. However, it requires surgical exploration over neck and is a relatively invasive method. On the contrary, the non-invasive method of embolization of the bleeder is possible and successful [35].

Neck Trauma

In neck injury patient, whether cervical spine stable or not is a crucial issue. While indicated, the patient should wear cervical collar for prevention from further cervical spine injury. In a case of severe trauma or multiple traumas, it is also necessary to pay attention to other concurrent injuries such as facial bone fracture, skull fracture with or without intracranial bleeding, clavicle fracture, rib fracture, extremities fracture, or intraabdomen bleeding which will complicate the whole condition and prolong the care time.

Hemorrhagic Diathesis

Hemorrhagic diathesis makes patient easy bleeding. Therefore, while patients with hemophila or other kind of hemorrhagic diatheisis, blood transfusion such as platelet or fresh frozen plasma for correction of bleeding tendency should be done. The support should be done initially and not delayed until the hematoma becomes more extensive.

Anticoagulant Usage

Once anticoagulant is suspiciously related to retropharyngeal hematoma, it is rationally to discontinuous the anticoagulant temporarily if no other contraindication. Component therapy is also applicable to patients with bleeding tendency for anticoagulant usage (as mentioned in the part of Hemorrhagic diathesis). Vitamin K support can be used in bleeding tendency because clotting factor II, IV, IX and X are Vitamin K dependent.

Neck Infection

The neck infection related retropharyngeal hematoma is often a severe condition that abscess is formation. The principle of management of such kind of neck infection is drainage of the abscess. It is reasonably to suspect that there is great vessels rupture. Be careful while exploration.

Foreign Body

The most important management is to remove foreign body. Because retropharyngeal hematoma existed, we should beware of whether the foreign body causes great vessels injury. In general, we can rule in or rule out this problem from CT scan. If great vessels are involved, angiography study should be performed and cardiovascular surgeon should be consulted before intervention. Possible risk should be informed.

Spontaneous

As mentioned before, except obvious trauma related retropharyngeal hematoma, an initial impression is either infection or tumor. Exploration should always be done for confirming the diagnosis and for relief of tension. Therefore, except of finding out any possible causes as we can, in spontaneous retropharyngeal hematoma, we should secure the airway and control the bleeding

Other Possible Causes

Specific management against the possible specific cause should also be taken. In the cases of parathyroid adenoma or cyst related retropharyngeal hematoma, excision is the way for diagnosis of the tumor and control the bleeding [67,68,69]. Surgical repair of the aneurysm is the key of control aneurysm rupture [5,72,73]. Epstein-Barr virus may induce hepatosplenomegaly and in consequence bleeding tendency occurs [78]. Management is the same as correct bleeding tendency.

Conclusion

Irrespective of any cause, retropharyngeal hematoma involves and compromises the aerodigestive tract and therefore is a life threatening problem. We should pay much attention to it and manage the near fatal condition carefully. As facing any patients in emergency, airway counts most. While securing airway or perform any other procedures, do not forget to protect the potentially fractured spine in trauma related cases. Finding out any possible cause of bleeding and correct it or repair it is the main steps we must take.

References

[1] Wong, Y. K. & Novotny, G. M. (1978). Retropharyngeal space - a review of anatomy, pathology, and clinical presentation. *J Otolaryngol, 7(6)*, 528-36.

[2] Hsu, T. Y., Tsai, T. C., et al. (2008). Near-fatal sore throat. *Lancet, 371(9618)*, 1136.

[3] Grodinsky, M. & Holyoke, E. A. (1938). The fasciae and fascial spaces of the head, neck and adjacent regions. *Am J Anat*, *63*, 367-408.

[4] Harnsberger, H. R. (1995). *Handbook of Head and Neck Imaging*. 2nd ed. St. Louis: Mosby, 89-104.

[5] Owens, D. E., Calcaterra, T. C., et al. (1975). Retropharyngeal hematoma. A complication of therapy with anticoagulants. *Arch Otolaryngol*, *101(9)*, 565-8.

[6] Coleman, J. A. Jr., & Johnson, J. T. (1986). Retropharyngeal hematoma: complication of cervical fracture. *Otolaryngol Head Neck Surg*, *94(3)*, 387-90.

[7] Al-Fallouji, H. K., Snow, D. G., et al. (1993). Spontaneous retropharyngeal haematoma: two cases and a review of the literature. *J Laryngol Otol*, *107(7)*, 649-50.

[8] Paleri, V., Maroju, R. S., et al. (2002). Spontaneous retro- and parapharyngeal haematoma caused by intrathyroid bleed. *J Laryngol Otol*, *116(10)*, 854-8.

[9] McLauchlan, C. A., Pidsley, R., et al. (1991). Minor trauma--major problem. Neck injuries, retropharyngeal haematoma and emergency airway management. *Arch Emerg Med*, *8(2)*, 135-9.

[10] Daniello, N. J. & Goldstein, S. I. (1994). Retropharyngeal hematoma secondary to minor blunt head and neck trauma. *Ear Nose Throat J*, *73(1)*, 41-3.

[11] Kette, F., Mergoni, P., et al. (2000). Delayed upper airway obstruction following a retropharyngeal haematoma after minor head trauma. *Eur J Emerg Med*, *7(4)*, 301-3.

[12] Tsai, K. J. & Huang, Y. C. (1999). Traumatic retropharyngeal hematoma: case report. *J Trauma*, *46(4)*, 715-6.

[13] Kochilas, X., Ali, A., et al. (2004). Retropharyngeal space swelling secondary to minor blunt head and neck trauma. *J Laryngol Otol*, *118(6)*, 465-7.

[14] Lazott, L. W., Ponzo, J. A., et al. (2007). Severe upper airway obstruction due to delayed retropharyngeal hematoma formation following blunt cervical trauma. *BMC Anesthesiol*, *7*, 2.

[15] Tsai, S. H., Hsu, C. W., et al. (2008). Traumatic retropharyngeal hematoma after a minor head injury. *J Trauma*, *64(2)*, 539.

[16] Mariani, P. J. (1990). Occipital condyle fracture presenting as retropharyngeal hematoma. *Ann Emerg Med*, *19(12)*, 1447-9.

[17] Freeman, B. J. & Behensky, H. (2005). Bilateral occipital condyle fractures leading to retropharyngeal haematoma and acute respiratory distress. *Injury*, *36(1)*, 207-12.

[18] De Wyngaert, R., Mulkens, T., et al. (2006). Bilateral occipital condylar fracture with associated haematomas. *Emerg Radiol*, *13(2)*, 79-82.

[19] Macnab, I. (1971). The whiplash syndrome. *Orthop Clin North Am*, *2(2)*, 389-403.

[20] Tenofsky, P. L., Porter, S. W., et al. (2000). Fatal airway compromise due to retropharyngeal hematoma after airbag deployment. *Am Surg*, *66(7)*, 692-4.

[21] Penning, L. (1981). Prevertebral hematoma in cervical spine injury: incidence and etiologic significance. *AJR Am J Roentgenol*, *136(3)*, 553-61.

[22] Smith, J. P., Morrissey, P., et al. (1988). Retropharyngeal hematomas. *J Trauma*, *28(4)*, 553-4.

[23] Kuhn, J. E. & Graziano, G. P. (1991). Airway compromise as a result of retropharyngeal hematoma following cervical spine injury. *J Spinal Disord*, *4(3)*, 264-9.

[24] Dingle, A. F., Clifford, K. M., et al. (1993). Retropharyngeal haematoma: a diagnosis for concern? *J Laryngol Otol*, *107(4)*, 356-8.

[25] Levine, R. J., Sanders, A. B., et al. (1995). Bilateral vocal cord paralysis following blunt trauma to the neck. *Ann Emerg Med*, *25(2)*, 253-5.

[26] Mitchell, R. O. & Heniford, B. T. (1995). Traumatic retropharyngeal hematoma--a cause of acute airway obstruction. *J Emerg Med*, *13(2)*, 165-7.

[27] Shaw, C. B., Bawa, R., et al. (1995). Traumatic retropharyngeal hematoma: a case report. *Otolaryngol Head Neck Surg*, *113(4)*, 485-8.

[28] Kelly, C. P., Haq, N., et al. (1995). Life-threatening retropharyngeal haematoma. *Injury*, *26(5)*, 339-40.

[29] O'Donnell, J. J., Birkinshaw, R., et al. (1997). Mechanical airway obstruction secondary to retropharyngeal haematoma. *Eur J Emerg Med*, *4(3)*, 166-8.

[30] Mazzon, D., Zanatta, P., et al. (1998). Upper airway obstruction by retropharyngeal hematoma after cervical spine trauma: report of a case treated with percutaneous dilational tracheostomy. *J Neurosurg Anesthesiol*, *10(4)*, 237-40.

[31] Cox, R. G. (1998). Retropharyngeal haematoma leading to airway obstruction in a child with closed head trauma. *Paediatr Anaesth*, *8(4)*, 353-6.

[32] Senthuran, S., Lim, S., et al. (1999). Life-threatening airway obstruction caused by a retropharyngeal haematoma. *Anaesthesia*, *54(7)*, 674-8.

[33] Sandooram, D., Chandramohan, A. R., et al. (2000). Retropharyngeal haematoma causing airway obstruction: a multidisciplinary challenge. *J Laryngol Otol*, *114(9)*, 706-8.

[34] El Kettani, C., Badaoui, R., et al. (2002). Traumatic retropharyngeal hematoma necessitating emergency intubation. *Anesthesiology*, *97(6)*, 1645-6.

[35] Van Velde, R., Sars, P. R., et al. (2002). Traumatic retropharyngeal haematoma treated by embolization of the thyrocervical trunk. *Eur J Emerg Med*, *9(2)*, 159-61.

[36] Shiratori, T., Hara, K., et al. (2003). Acute airway obstruction secondary to retropharyngeal hematoma. *J Anesth*, *17(1)*, 46-8.

[37] Suzuki, T., Imai, H., et al. (2004). Fatal retropharyngeal haematoma secondary to blunt trauma. *Injury*, *35(10)*, 1059-63.

[38] O'Neill, J. V., Toomey, J. M., et al. (1977). Retropharyngeal hematoma secondary to minor blunt trauma in the elderly patient. *J Otolaryngol, 6(1)*, 43-6.

[39] Bray, G. & Nugent, D. (1986). Hemorrhage involving the upper airway in hemophilia. *Clin Pediatr (Phila), 25(9)*, 436-9.

[40] Macik, B. G., Hohneker, J., et al. (1989). Use of recombinant activated factor VII for treatment of a retropharyngeal hemorrhage in a hemophilic patient with a high titer inhibitor. *Am J Hematol, 32(3)*, 232-4.

[41] Harper, M., Obolensky, L., et al. (2007). A case of acute upper and lower airway obstruction due to retropharyngeal haemorrhage secondary to acquired haemophilia A. *Anaesthesia, 62(6)*, 627-30.

[42] Macik, B. G., Hohneker, J., et al. (1989). Use of recombinant activated factor VII for treatment of a retropharyngeal hemorrhage in a hemophilic patient with a high titer inhibitor. *Am J Hematol, 32(3)*, 232-4.

[43] Sinert, R. & Scalea, T. (1994). Retropharyngeal and bowel hematomas in an anticoagulated patient. *Acad Emerg Med, 1(1)*, 67-72.

[44] Carmody, T. J. & Wergowske, G. L. (1983). Retropharyngeal abscess and hematoma in an elderly woman following esophagoscopy and endotracheal intubation. *J Am Geriatr Soc, 31(8)*, 499-500.

[45] Thatcher, J. & George, D. (1987). Retropharyngeal hematoma as a new cause of acute upper airway obstruction in rheumatoid arthritis. *J Rheumatol, 14(6)*, 1172-3.

[46] Bapat, V. N., Brown, K., et al. (2002). Retropharyngeal hematoma--a rare complication of anticoagulant therapy. *Eur J Cardiothorac Surg, 21(1)*, 117-8.

[47] Chiti-Batelli, S., Vaz, F., et al. (2005). Traumatic retropharyngeal haematoma in an anticoagulated patient: Case report and proposal for a clinical protocol. *Acta Otolaryngol, 125(4)*, 443-5.

[48] Akoglu, E., Seyfeli, E., et al. (2008). Retropharyngeal hematoma as a complication of anticoagulation therapy. *Ear Nose Throat J, 87(3)*, 156-9.

[49] Srivastava, S. & Solanki, T. (2008). Retropharyngeal haematoma - an unusual bleeding site in an anticoagulated patient: a case report. *Cases J, 1(1)*, 294.

[50] Genovesi, M. G. & Simmons, D. H. (1975). Airway obstruction due to spontaneous retropharyngeal hemorrhage. *Chest, 68(6)*, 840-2.

[51] Rosenbaum, L., Thurman, P., et al. (1979). Upper airway obstruction as a complication of oral anticoagulation therapy. Report of three cases. *Arch Intern Med*, *139(10)*, 1151-3.

[52] Bloom, D. C., Haegen, T., et al. (2003). Anticoagulation and spontaneous retropharyngeal hematoma. *J Emerg Med*, *24(4)*, 389-94.

[53] Gonzalez-Garcia, R., Schoendorff, G., et al. (2006). Upper airway obstruction by sublingual hematoma: a complication of anticoagulation therapy with acenocoumarol. *Am J Otolaryngol*, *27(2)*, 129-32.

[54] Myssiorek, D. & Shalmi, C. (1989). Traumatic retropharyngeal hematoma. *Arch Otolaryngol Head Neck Surg*, *115(9)*, 1130-2.

[55] Chin, K. W., Sercarz, J. A., et al. (1998). Spontaneous cervical hemorrhage with near-complete airway obstruction. *Head Neck*, *20(4)*, 350-3.

[56] Vakees, Y. S., Hashemi, K., et al. (2000). Retropharyngeal haematoma after blunt trauma. *J Accid Emerg Med*, *17(6)*, 430.

[57] Miller, R., Collison, P., et al. (2006). Spontaneous retropharyngeal hemorrhage causing airway obstruction: a case report with a review of the literature. *S D Med*, *59(7)*, 295-7, 299.

[58] McNair, T. J. (1967). *Hamilton Bailey's emergency surgery*, 8th edition. Bristol, 264.

[59] Hays, H. (1964). Retropharyngeal hemorrhage: A fatal case. *Tex State J Med*, *60*,904-905.

[60] Clark, W. G. & Monks, C. J. (1969). Retropharyngeal haematoma. *J Laryngol Otol*, *83(10)*, 1039-42.

[61] Ophir, D. & Bartal, N. (1988). Retropharyngeal hematoma following fish-bone ingestion. *Ear Nose Throat J*, *67(7)*, 528-30.

[62] Weiqan Chang Hsueh-Yu Li (2000). Retropharyngeal hematoma following chicken-bone misswallowing - case report. *J Taiwan Otolaryngol Head Neck Surg*, *35(6)*, 394-397.

[63] Schroder, K. E. & Mair, I. W. (1978). Spontaneous haematoma in the head and neck. *J Laryngol Otol*, *92(3)*, 215-21.

[64] Rotter, N., Jager, L., et al. (2008). Spontaneous retropharyngeal hematoma: a rare differential diagnosis of acute dysphagia. *HNO*, *56(9)*, 981-4.

[65] Singh, A., Ofo, E., et al. (2008). Spontaneous retropharyngeal haematoma: a case report. *J Med Case Reports*, *2*, 8.

[66] Pickett, G. E., Sekhon, L. H., et al. (2006). Complications with cervical arthroplasty. *J Neurosurg Spine*, *4(2)*, 98-105.

[67] Ku, P., Scott, P., et al. (1998). Spontaneous retropharyngeal haematoma in a parathyroid adenoma. *Aust N Z J Surg*, *68(8)*, 619-21.

[68] Nito, T., Miyajima, C., et al. (2007). Parathyroid adenoma causing spontaneous cervical hematoma: a case report. *Acta Otolaryngol*, *Suppl(559)*, 160-3.

[69] Taniguchi, I., Maeda, T., et al. (2003). Spontaneous retropharyngeal hematoma of a parathyroid cyst: report of a case. *Surg Today*, *33(5)*, 354-7.

[70] Koulouris, G., Pianta, M., et al. (2006). The 'sentinel clot' sign in spontaneous retropharyngeal hematoma secondary to parathyroid apoplexy. *Ear Nose Throat J*, *85(9)*, 606-8.

[71] Thomas, M. D., Torres, A., et al. (1991). Life-threatening cervico-mediastinal haematoma after carotid sinus massage. *J Laryngol Otol*, *105(5)*, 381-3.

[72] Sabra, O., Sabri, A., et al. (2006). Airway obstruction secondary to thoracic aortic aneurysm leak. A case report. *Eur Arch Otorhinolaryngol*, *263(12)*, 1144-6.

[73] Newton, A. I. (2006). Spontaneous retropharyngeal hematoma: an unusual presentation of thoracic aortic dissection. *J Emerg Med*, *31(1)*, 45-8.

[74] Stewart, R. W., Hardjasudarma, M., et al. (1995). Fatal outcome of jugular vein cannulation. *South Med J*, *88(11)*, 1159-60.

[75] Higa, K., Hirata, K., et al. (2006). Retropharyngeal hematoma after stellate ganglion block: Analysis of 27 patients reported in the literature. *Anesthesiology*, *105(6)*, 1238-45; discussion 5A-6A.

[76] Okuda, Y., Urabe, K., et al. (2003). Retropharyngeal or cervicomediastinal haematomas following stellate ganglion block. *Eur J Anaesthesiol*, *20(9)*, 757-9.

[77] Munoz, A., Fischbein, N. J., et al. (2001). Spontaneous retropharyngeal hematoma: diagnosis by mr imaging. *AJNR Am J Neuroradiol*, *22(6)*, 1209-11.

[78] Jones, T. M., Owen, G. O., et al. (1996). Spontaneous retropharyngeal haematoma attributable to Epstein-Barr virus infection. *J Laryngol Otol*, *110(11)*, 1075-7.

[79] Draper, M. R., Sandhu, G., et al. (1999). Retropharyngeal haematoma causing acute airway obstruction--first presentation of metastatic carcinoma. *J Laryngol Otol*, *113(3)*, 258-9.

[80] Wholey, M. H., Bruwer, A. J., et al. (1958). The lateral roentgenogram of the neck; with comments on the atlanto-odontoid-basion relationship. *Radiology*, *71(3)*, 350-6.
[81] White, P., Seymour, R. & Powell, N. (1999). MRI assessment of the prevertebral soft tissues in the acute cervical spine trauma. *Br J Radiol*, *72*, 818-823.
[82] Capps, R. B. (1934). Multiple parathyroid tumors with massive mediastinal and subcutaneous hemorrhage. *Am J Med Sci*, *188(6)*, 800-805.
[83] Sandor, F. & Cooke, R. T. (1964). Spontaneous Cervico-Mediastinal Haematoma. *Br J Surg*, *51*, 682-6.

Index

A

B

D

E

F

G

H

I

Q

R

S

T

U

V

W

X